HELPING YOUR HEALTH
WITH
POINTED PRESSURE THERAPY

HELPING YOUR HEALTH
WITH
POINTED PRESSURE THERAPY

ROY E. BEAN, N.D.

PARKER PUBLISHING COMPANY, INC.
WEST NYACK, N.Y.

Library of Congress Cataloging in Publication Data

Bean, Roy E
    Helping your health with pointed pressure therapy.

    Includes index.
    1. Massage. I. Title.
RM721.B38   615'.822   75-12855

*To my family
and especially
to my mother*

ACKNOWLEDGEMENTS

I want to thank my wife Esther and my daughter Donna for their hours of compiling and typing. I also want to thank Robert Gresens for his invaluable illustrations.

WHAT THIS BOOK CAN DO FOR YOU

Every organ and its associated problems has at least one response area. Response areas are sensitive spots that are located all over the body. They will only be tender if a problem exists. Once the problem is gone the tenderness disappears.

In this book we will concern ourselves with a system of healing which deals with a unique and special type of massage which we call Pointed Pressure Therapy. By applying this pressure therapy to the response areas you can restore each and every organ and their systems to their original healthy state. Health is only *a little pressure on the right spot* away.

While this is not a cure-all, it does promise relief and often the complete remission of many common problems. You will be amazed at the results you will have in ridding yourself of such common problems as sinus trouble, backache, headache, and gas. Crippling diseases such as arthritis yield to Pointed Pressure Therapy. Your body has remarkable recuperative powers but usually it requires some help. You can give it that help by mastering this massage technique.

Pointed Pressure Therapy can be used by the physician and layman alike. Without the use of needles or drugs, you can relieve hundreds of common disorders and alleviate much pain. All you need to do is study the charts and treatments outlined in this book. You will then be able to apply the pressure massage required to accomplish wonders for yourself and others.

This method of pain relief and disease control is over 6,000 years old. Wise men of the centuries have continued its use in many forms under many names such as reflexology, and zone therapy. It is similar to the Oriental technique of acupuncture, though completely without the use of needles. Its origin, development, use and theories of how it works are explained in this book in the hope that some of the mystery surrounding it can be explained and thereby pointed pressure therapy can become a useful therapeutic system for you.

Roy E. Bean, N.D.

Table of Contents

Chapter 6   How to Treat Stomach Problems *(Cont.)*

Chapter 15   Quick Relief For Minor Ailments *(Cont.)*

HELPING YOUR HEALTH
WITH
POINTED PRESSURE THERAPY

chapter 1

The Origin of
Pointed Pressure
Massage and
Theories of
How It Works

Thousands of years ago man discovered that there was a connection between certain disorders of the body and a tenderness on certain areas of the body. How and when this discovery was made is not known but its use dates back over 6000 years. It has been suggested that the first attempt to attribute healing powers to this massage resulted from a sudden remission of an acute attack of appendicitis following a bruise on the response area located on the bottom of the foot. Another suggestion explains its discovery by the sudden relief of stammering in a warrior who had been shot in the back of the neck with an arrow. Proponents of acupuncture find this explanation suitable in the use of needles.

A more recent view is that through the use of general back rubbing massage, certain unexplained tender spots were found to be present in recognizable disorders. By applying localized, deep penetrating pressure massage the disorders mysteriously vanished. Many other theories have been advanced regarding its discovery but no one really knows how or when it was actually discovered.

It has been called many different names during the ages and has been used successfully by skilled practitioners over a period of thousands of years. It has also been tried by some very superficially without success because they were ill advised as to how to apply the massage effectively. In this book we will outline a method of applying the Pointed Pressure Massage which will insure results when applied properly. By studying the charts and case histories you will become familiar with the methods involved and what you can expect to bring results for you.

THEORIES ABOUT HOW IT WORKS

There are many theories about how this type of massage works. We will explain several of the most common ones here in an effort to help you understand more about this ancient mode of healing.

I. NERVE STIMULATION THEORY

This theory, often called Nerve Blockage, is a commonly advanced theory as to how Pressure Massage works. With this theory a suitable means of connection between the disorder and the response area is assumed. The pressure on the response area is thought to transmit repair messages to the brain center causing the body to mobilize its forces.

II. LYMPH THEORY

Since the lymph vessels provide drainage channels into the lymph nodes for toxic or malignant products, it is assumed that pressure on the appropriate areas will enhance their function thereby restoring the proper chemical balance in the body.

III. CIRCULATION THEORY

The entire body is dependent on the circulatory system for its survival. Food products for nourishment and waste products are both transported with this system. Partial blockage or impaired circulation are assumed to be the key factors in waste removal problems. Improved nourishment is seen as a result of Pointed Pressure Massage.

IV. CRYSTALS IMPEDING
NERVE TRANSFER THEORY

Nerve endings are presumed to be rendered unable to transmit their impulses because of a build up of a crystalline deposit which blocks the pathway. Pointed Pressure Massage is credited with the breaking up of these crystals and thus restoring the normal flow of the impulses again.

V. ELECTRIC POTENTIAL THEORY

It has long been held that a difference in electrical potential in various parts of the body constituted a corresponding malfunction in another part of the body. Recently the Oriental scientists have been able to demonstrate with newly designed instruments of the sophisticated space age technology that this actually does exist. More research is being conducted in this field to determine causes and possible means of correcting the imbalance. Many of the questions as to how this relates to Pressure Massage may find answers in this program.

VI. REFLEXES

A reflex action is a response to a sensory stimulus initiated somewhere in the body to cause a reaction somewhere else in the body usually occurring without immediate involvement of the brain. The reflex arc consists of five components: a sensory receptor, a sensory neuron, one or more internuncial neurons, a motor neuron and an effector such as a gland or a muscle. Since this is a clinically demonstrable process it has failed to explain the results of Pointed Pressure Massage in its entirety because certain response areas do not contain the reflexes and yet work as well as those which do.

VII. PSYCHOLOGICAL

Many have tried to explain the results as merely the power of suggestion. I have been able to completely rule out this by experimentation in the animal world. Anyone experienced in working with horses knows the value of applying a twitch around the upper lip of the animal when medical attention is required for an injury or disease. Pain can be completely controlled for a period of time by keeping the twitch on during the treatment. A similar form of temporary anesthesia in the animal world is present in the carrying of kittens by the nape of the neck by the mother.

VIII. VITAL FORCES THEORY

An attempt to explain Pointed Pressure Massage by the mystical vital forces of Oriental writings fails to establish any biological basis for its explanation. The success of the massage is primarily the result of adequate attention to proper use of existing techniques.

IX. COUNTER IRRITATION

The human body has the ability to speed up repair when it receives any insult to its equilibrium. Many assume that Pressure Massage does slightly insult the body and therefore as an irritation summons the defences into action. It is true that the body can be spurred into action by externally applied forces. Some can be demonstrated clinically and thus give credence to this view.

SUMMARY

The above theories are just theories. They all have some merit in explaining the results but none of them can actually be used as a technical explanation of the manner in which the actual healing is brought about. We do not know how it works only that it does and has for scores of people over the centuries.

chapter 2

How To Apply
Pointed Pressure
Massage

Nature provided a simple method of massage in the form of walking barefooted over the uneven surface of the ground. For general relaxation this will provide a means of massage but for specific problems a more direct approach will be necessary.

Pointed Pressure Massage differs from general massage such as back rubbing in that the massage is directed at a specific location for a specific length of time. The specific location is called a response area. This is an area about the size of a pea which is known to be responsive to external pressure and is directly associated with an organ or pain center. These areas appear over the entire body but are concentrated on the bottom of the feet and on the palm of the hands. Tenderness in these areas is present only when there is a malfunction or pain in the body. The specific length of time is usually nine minutes at each location every other day until the soreness on the response area is alleviated. At this time the condition will have been corrected. The pressure in the area cited must be great enough to cause some discomfort if the massage is to be effective. An exact location of the response area is not critical when digital or mechanical pressure massage is used since the necessary points will be covered by following the general location on the charts in this book.

STEPS IN APPLYING
THIS METHOD OF MASSAGE

First you will have to study the charts in Chapter 3. In that chapter there will be an explanation of each chart which will help you understand how to use them. Note the exact response area for specific organs or problems and their corresponding zones. This is very important in helping you picture the location of the organs and the response areas for each one. Once you have familiarized yourself with the charts you will be able to locate the response areas for any specific problem you may have which will be described in this book.

After comparing your symptoms, aches and pains with those described in this book you will be able to apply pressure massage to the proper response area. This is a very simple technique. I would first suggest that you seat yourself in a comfortable chair. If the response area to be massaged is on your foot or leg, that foot or leg must be rested on the thigh of the other leg so that you will be able to easily reach it with both hands.

Hold the foot or leg with one hand and apply pressure massage to the response area as shown on the charts, with the other. This may be done with the fingers, thumbs, knuckles or with a mechanical aid as described in Chapter 3.

At first you may have to hunt a little for the specific area as you familiarize yourself with the response areas. This isn't really very hard and doesn't take long because if you apply enough pressure properly, the response area will hurt. I believe this is the beauty of the technique. Only those response areas for specific problems which afflict you will be sore. Once the problem is gone they will no longer be sore.

Once you locate the tender spot and begin to apply the pressure, be sure the "soreness" is still felt throughout the treatment. If it disappears you may not be pressing hard enough or you may not be on the response area any longer. Find the "sore spot" again and continue the pressure.

The exact type of massage used here is important. It must be in a circular fashion with penetrating pressure which does not rub the outer skin but rather massages the subdermal layers of the skin and tissues thoroughly for nine minutes each treatment.

Response areas on the hands, arms, ears or face are also easy to apply pressure massage to because you can reach them with one hand while sitting in a comfortable position. Those on the back and spine are not as easy to apply pressure massage to. In some cases you may need someone — a spouse, a relative or a trusted friend — to apply the pressure for you or you may need to use a mechanical aid such as one described for the back in Chapter 3.

In cases where it is not feasible to use the above methods, the use of rubber bands can be very effective. This consists of placing rubber bands on the joints of each finger or toes as specified. In an acute case, the bands should be placed on the first joint of all fingers or toes (the joints closest to the nail). In chronic cases, place the bands just below the second joint of the fingers or toes daily. In both cases the bands should be wrapped tightly and remain on for nine full minutes for the best results. *Never* leave them on over 11 minutes at a time because this will impair circulation!

Another very simple means of applying the pressure is to clamp wooden clothes pins on the ends of the fingers or toes over the nails for nine minutes as a general application of this therapy.

The use of the rubber bands on the toes and fingers as well as the clothes pins is recommended for those who have impaired use of their hands or feet such as in arthritis.

SUMMARY OF HOW TO USE AND
APPLY PRESSURE MASSAGE

1. Study the charts in Chapter 3.

2. Apply pressure with the thumb or a mechanical aid on the general location of the response area to find out "where it hurts."

3. When the problem is more obscure, apply pressure massage to the entire palm of the hand or sole of the foot noting the tender areas. Massage these "sore spots" nine minutes each treatment.

4. In cases where pressure must be applied in other ways use rubber bands or clothes pins.

chapter 3

How To Spot The Key Response Areas

To help you understand Pointed Pressure Therapy and how to use it effectively you must study and understand the charts of the body, the zones, the organs, and the response areas to the organs.

UNDERSTANDING CHART 1
(ZONES)

Study Chart 1 carefully. You will see that the body is divided up into 5 zones on each side. The center of the body is zone 1 for the right and left side. By looking at this chart and reading this explanation of the zones, you will become acquainted with these zones and have a better understanding of the human body.

Note: Although the following charts depict a male figure, you may apply Pointed Pressure Therapy at the same points on both men and women.

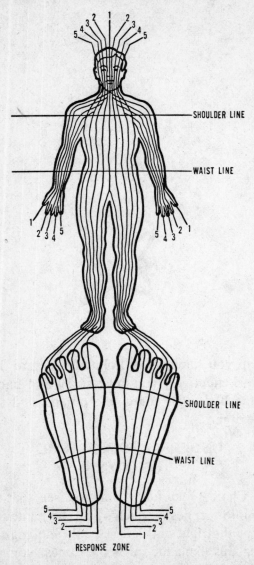

CHART 1

Zone 1 extends from the tip of the thumb, straight up to the top of the head, down through the nostrils and then through the center of the body to the big toe. It includes the stomach, the nasal passage, the palate, many of the glands, the esophagus, spine, the uterus, bladder, anus, sex organs and the heart on the left side. Any problem with these organs can be treated by applying pressure massage to the response areas for the organs in zone 1, whether on the face, arms, legs or feet.

Zone 2 extends from the index finger up to the head and down to the second toe. It includes the eyes, the sinuses, many of the glands, the lungs, bronchial tubes, the tonsils, stomach, the heart and pancreas on the left side. Here you can see that some of the organs such as the stomach are also found in zone 2 as well as in 1. In this case the response area will be bigger and be located over both zones. If you have trouble with any of these organs their response areas will be easy to find if you look in zone 2.

The third zone extends from the middle finger, up to the head and down to the middle toe. It includes the eyes, some glands, the lungs, the kidneys, the stomach on the left side, the appendix, the liver, and the gall bladder on the right side.

Zone 4 begins at the tip of the 4th finger, up to the head and down to the 4th toe. It includes the appendix, liver, ileo-cecal valve on the right side only; the shoulders, ears, and lungs; and the spleen on the left side only.

The fifth zone extends from the little finger, up to the head and down to the little toe. It includes the liver on the right side only, the ears and the back of the neck. If you have any problem connected with your liver, pressure massage in this zone as well as in zone 4 will eliminate it.

All of these zones run evenly over the entire body — the arms, legs, hands and feet. The tip of the foot corresponds with the head while the back of the foot corresponds with the end of the spine.

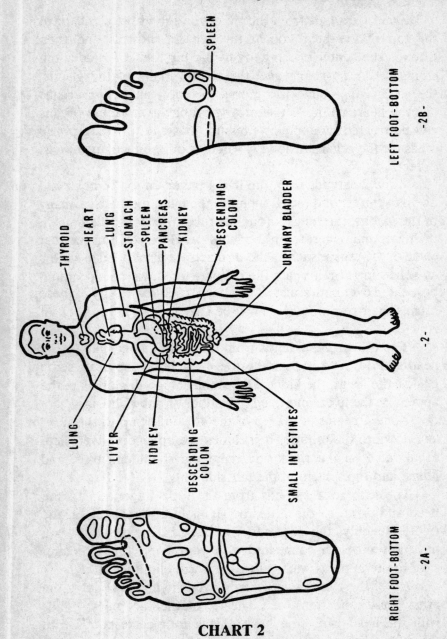

SPLEEN

LEFT FOOT-BOTTOM
-2B-

THYROID
HEART
LUNG
STOMACH
SPLEEN
PANCREAS
KIDNEY
DESCENDING COLON
URINARY BLADDER

LUNG
LIVER
KIDNEY
DESCENDING COLON
SMALL INTESTINES

-2-

RIGHT FOOT-BOTTOM
-2A-

CHART 2

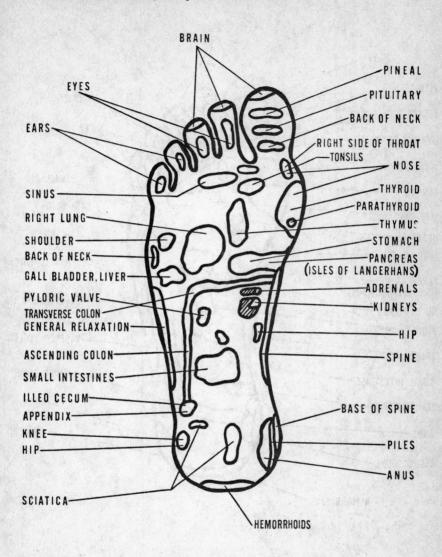

BRAIN

PINEAL

PITUITARY

EYES

BACK OF NECK

EARS

RIGHT SIDE OF THROAT

TONSILS

NOSE

THYROID

SINUS

PARATHYROID

RIGHT LUNG

THYMUS

SHOULDER

STOMACH

BACK OF NECK

PANCREAS

GALL BLADDER, LIVER

(ISLES OF LANGERHANS)

ADRENALS

PYLORIC VALVE

KIDNEYS

TRANSVERSE COLON

GENERAL RELAXATION

HIP

ASCENDING COLON

SPINE

SMALL INTESTINES

ILLEO CECUM

APPENDIX

BASE OF SPINE

KNEE

HIP

PILES

ANUS

SCIATICA

HEMORRHOIDS

RIGHT FOOT-BOTTOM

-2A-

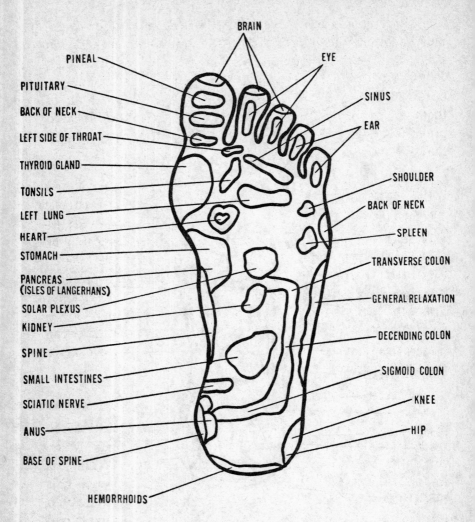

BRAIN

PINEAL

PITUITARY

BACK OF NECK

LEFT SIDE OF THROAT

THYROID GLAND

TONSILS

LEFT LUNG

HEART

STOMACH

PANCREAS
(ISLES OF LANGERHANS)

SOLAR PLEXUS

KIDNEY

SPINE

SMALL INTESTINES

SCIATIC NERVE

ANUS

BASE OF SPINE

HEMORRHOIDS

EYE

SINUS

EAR

SHOULDER

BACK OF NECK

SPLEEN

TRANSVERSE COLON

GENERAL RELAXATION

DECENDING COLON

SIGMOID COLON

KNEE

HIP

LEFT FOOT — BOTTOM

- 2B -

Many organs lie in several or all of the zones. For example the brain, the intestines and the sinuses all lie in each zone. Specific parts of these organs lie in a specific zone.

Organs like the ears and kidneys, which are found on both sides of the body will have response areas on both of the hands and feet. The appendix and heart which are located predominately on one side will have response areas only on that side.

UNDERSTANDING CHART 2
(ORGANS-ZONES)

As you look at Charts 2, 2A, 2B, you will see exactly where the organs are in the body and the corresponding zones they lie in. Also the response areas for these organs that are located on the bottom of your feet are shown. If you have a problem with digestion for example, you would massage the response areas for the organs of the digestive system in their corresponding zones. You always work in the zone where the organ is attached to the body. The entrance and exit of the organ are the most important areas to massage for treatment.

UNDERSTANDING CHART 3

Now look at Chart 3. Besides the response areas located on the feet there are response areas all over the body. Many times the hands or feet are easier to massage but nevertheless important response areas are also on the arms and legs. This chart shows some of the common problems and their associated response areas. These areas correspond to the zones explained under Chart 1.

UNDERSTANDING CHART 4
(FACIAL)

Now let's look at Chart 4. The head and neck area contain many very important response areas. It is a relatively

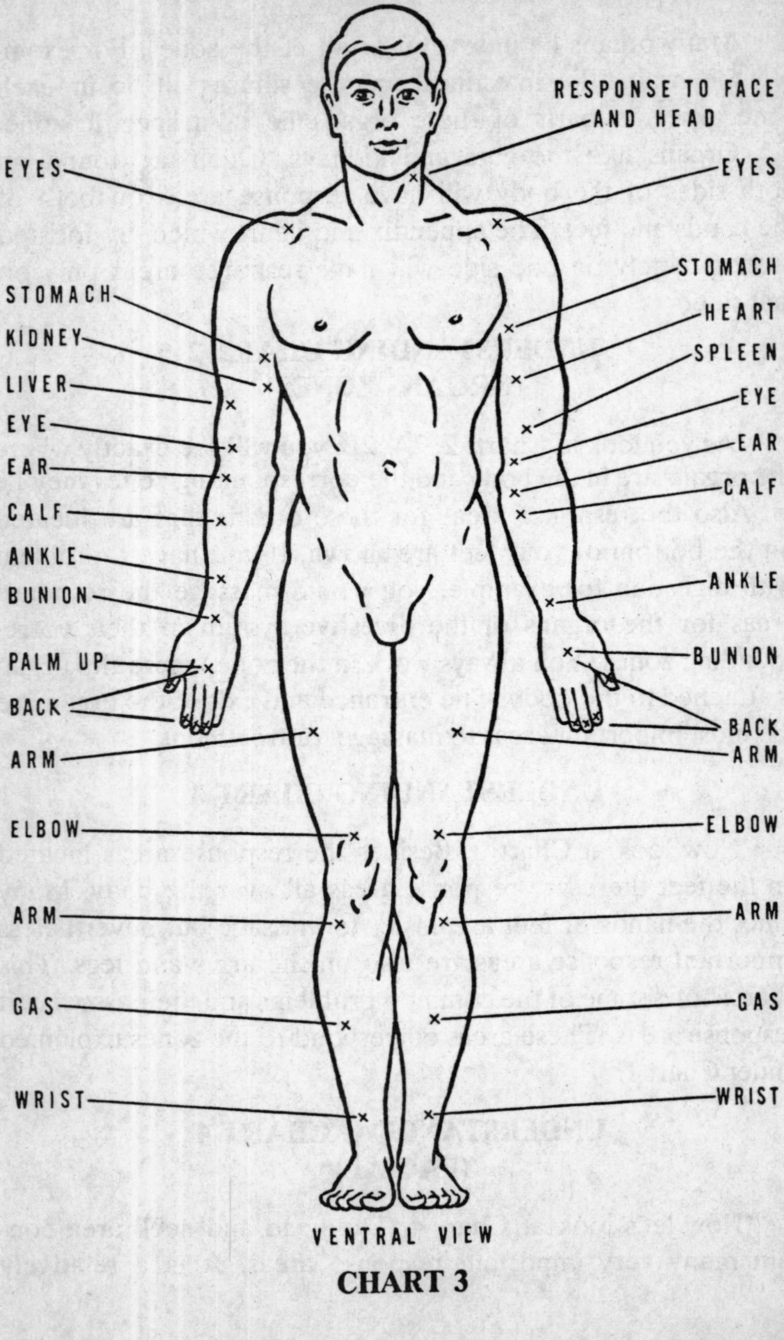

RESPONSE TO FACE
AND HEAD

EYES   EYES

                                                  STOMACH
STOMACH   HEART
KIDNEY   SPLEEN
LIVER   EYE
EYE   EAR
EAR   CALF
CALF

ANKLE   ANKLE
BUNION
                                                  BUNION
PALM UP
BACK   BACK
ARM   ARM

ELBOW   ELBOW

ARM   ARM

GAS   GAS

WRIST   WRIST

VENTRAL VIEW

CHART 3

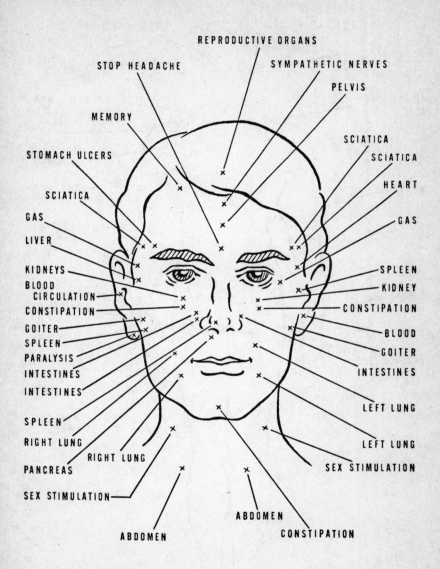

REPRODUCTIVE ORGANS
STOP HEADACHE
SYMPATHETIC NERVES
PELVIS
MEMORY
SCIATICA
STOMACH ULCERS
SCIATICA
HEART
SCIATICA
GAS
GAS
LIVER
KIDNEYS
SPLEEN
BLOOD CIRCULATION
KIDNEY
CONSTIPATION
CONSTIPATION
GOITER
BLOOD
SPLEEN
GOITER
PARALYSIS
INTESTINES
INTESTINES
INTESTINES
SPLEEN
LEFT LUNG
RIGHT LUNG
LEFT LUNG
RIGHT LUNG
PANCREAS
SEX STIMULATION
SEX STIMULATION
ABDOMEN
ABDOMEN
CONSTIPATION

CHART 4

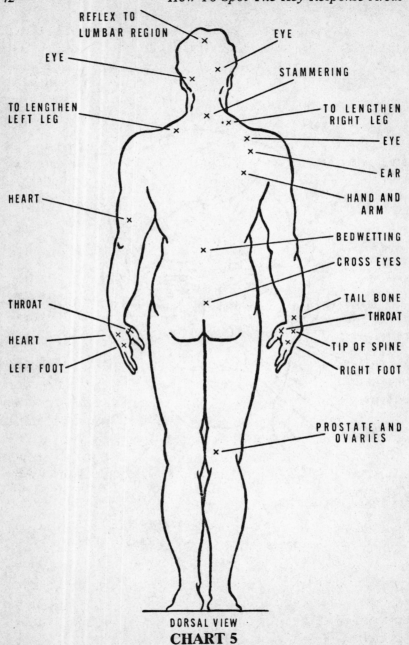

REFLEX TO
LUMBAR REGION

EYE

EYE

STAMMERING

TO LENGTHEN
LEFT LEG

TO LENGTHEN
RIGHT LEG

EYE

EAR

HAND AND
ARM

HEART

BEDWETTING

CROSS EYES

TAIL BONE

THROAT

THROAT

HEART

TIP OF SPINE

LEFT FOOT

RIGHT FOOT

PROSTATE AND
OVARIES

DORSAL VIEW
CHART 5

easy area to apply pressure massage to and can bring results that can't be compared with. Three very important problems have response areas included in the facial area. They are headaches, constipation and paralysis. It will be helpful to study this chart and learn these areas.

UNDERSTANDING CHART 5

This chart is the back view of the body and corresponds with Chart 3. It shows more response areas for various organs and problems.

UNDERSTANDING CHART 6
(FEET)

Besides the response areas on the bottom of the foot there are many important ones on the sides, back and top of the foot. This chart includes these response areas.

MECHANICAL AIDS

Many devices have been developed which make it possible to apply the pressure required for this form of therapy without using the thumbs or fingers. This is important to the Doctor since his hands are usually required to do other things in addition to the pressure massage in treating a patient. It is also important to anyone who doesn't have a strong enough grip to apply the proper amount of pressure needed in the treatment.

These aids come in three basic forms. The first form is any device with a blunted point which can be held in the hand and used to press firmly on the response areas. It may look something like the one in Figure A.

The second form has either a blunted point attached to a base which can be used on the floor for the foot to be pressed against or something that is round such as a ball or cylinder which the foot is rolled over. See Figure B.

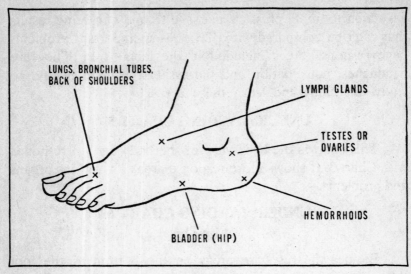

LUNGS, BRONCHIAL TUBES,
BACK OF SHOULDERS

LYMPH GLANDS

TESTES OR
OVARIES

HEMORRHOIDS

BLADDER (HIP)

RIGHT FOOT

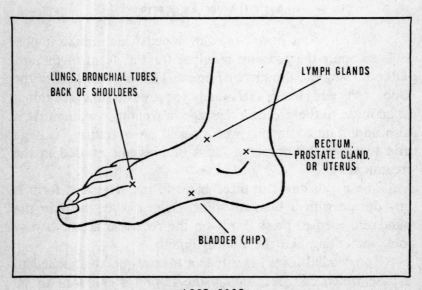

LUNGS, BRONCHIAL TUBES,
BACK OF SHOULDERS

LYMPH GLANDS

RECTUM,
PROSTATE GLAND,
OR UTERUS

BLADDER (HIP)

LEFT FOOT

CHART 6

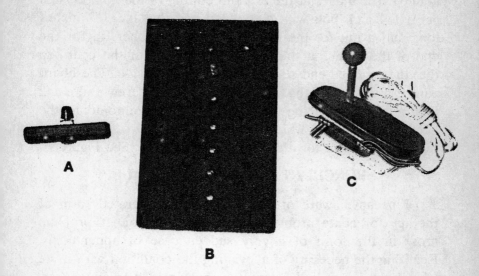

A

B

C

The third form is a blunted point or a rounded object attached to a vibrator in such a manner that the vibrating point can be pressed against the response area. See Figure C.

Besides these specific pressure applicators there are many general vibrating-stretching devices which are beneficial. Your doctor whether he be a Naturopath, Chiropractor or an Osteopath would be in a position to help you decide which ones would best suit your needs.

If you need to apply pressure to a response area that is on the back or spine or on an area that you can't reach you may need someone else to apply the pressure for you. When this is not possible I would suggest that you make a mechanical aid of your own. An adjustable mechanical aid on the wall will come in very handy for those response areas on your back. Here is how you make one of your own.

Get a foot long board that is 3/4 inch thick and 6 inches wide and cut a 3/8 inch slot through the middle of it. Leave about 1 to 2 inches at the top and bottom of the board. Then get a 1/4 inch bolt with a rounded end that is 2-1/2 inches long and a nut for the bolt as well as a rubber tip for the end of the bolt. Put the bolt in the bottom of the board so that the rounded end sticks out on the front side. The board can be mounted on the wall with a 1/4 inch screw and a 1/2 inch washer. Loosening the screw will allow you to adjust the height of the board which changes the height of the bolt to the proper height for a specific response area. See Figure C.

BUNCHING — A NEW TECHNIQUE

I became aware of a need for an accelerated form of therapy for acute problems as a young doctor. A problem arose in the form of a very sudden case of appendicitis. Realizing the necessity of alleviating the condition with haste to stop the appendix from rupturing, I decided to apply pressure massage in more than one way concurrently to see if the results could be achieved faster than could normally be expected. The results were so dramatic that I began using this technique for speedy results when time was really important. This has thus developed into a unique approach which I have called "Bunching."

This technique involves continuous pressure massage by the use of rubber bands on the joints of the fingers. These must be wrapped tightly and remain on for nine minutes. Clothes pins on the tips of the toes for nine minutes is the second step in bunching. Digital Pointed Pressure Massage on the specific response areas on the bottom of the feet or on the hands, legs or arms and finally biting your tongue completes the technique. All of this must be done at the same time or in rapid succession. To bite your tongue properly, stick it out about 1/2 inch and bite down on it for nine minutes at a time. This technique is a most effective therapy when acute problems such as migraine headaches arise.

chapter 4

How To Relieve
Those Aching Joints

Joints are places of union between two or more bones. They are grouped three ways according to the degree of movement they permit and serve the dual purpose of bearing weight and providing motion. They are formed to provide stability. We are interested mainly in the freely movable joints because this is where most problems and aches begin.

In many joints there is a sac with fluid in it. These sacs are called bursae. They help the gliding of muscles or tendons over bones or ligaments and without them friction would develop.

BURSITIS

One common disorder of the joints occurring in the bursae is called Bursitis which is an inflammation of these

sacs that usually results from excess strain or tension placed
upon the bursae. The most common area for this to occur is
in the bursa of the shoulder joint. When this occurs movement of the shoulder is painful and if it persists, the muscles
eventually atrophy or degenerate, causing the shoulder to
become stiff. Inflammation of the bursae in the elbows, knees
and ankles can cause similar problems which you can remove
by applying Pointed Pressure Massage to the bottom of your
foot.

As you look at Figure 2A you see the response area for the
shoulder is on the outside of the bottom of the foot just below
the joint at the base of the little toe.

Seat yourself comfortably in position so you can hold your
foot and apply pressure with your thumb on the bottom of the
foot. Considerable pressure must be applied for nine minutes.
Treatment should be twice weekly until the tenderness is gone
and the condition is relieved. Vigorous massage (make it hurt a
little) will bring speedy results but since some people bruise
easier than others you should start with only moderate pressure
and then gradually increase it for the greatest benefit.

A CASE OF BURSITIS

Mrs. D. began having pain in her shoulder area on the
right side. She had been on a bowling team for years but was
forced to quit because of the pain. She had delayed any treatment except for home rubbing compounds because she thought
that surgery was the only solution.

My examination revealed the extreme tenderness of the
response area for the shoulder directly under the little toe, on
the bottom of her foot. I began a series of Pointed Pressure
Massage treatments on this area which continued for twenty
weeks. At first she had only temporary reduction in the pain.
This lasted for less than eight hours after each treatment. After
the fifth week she began to notice the severity of the pain was

greatly reduced around the clock. In another ten weeks she was well enough to resume bowling, but continued treatments another five weeks for complete recovery.

ANOTHER CASE OF BURSITIS

Mrs. L. had smoked heavily for years and was also a heavy coffee drinker. These two habits had made her body deficient in Vitamin C and caused her to be easy prey to problems with the joints and connective tissue.

She had enjoyed tennis but was suddenly forced to quit because of a pain in her shoulder that would not go away. When this was diagnosed as Bursitis she was afraid surgery would eventually be required. She came to my office for help in controlling the pain. I explained my reluctance to apply Pointed Pressure Massage unless she could rid herself of the smoking and coffee drinking. I felt we could definitely help with pressure massage but only if she cooperated in removing the factors contributing to her problem.

We agreed to one treatment to reduce the immediate pain and then left the possibility of future treatments conditioned on the decision regarding coffee and smoking. You see the caffein and nicotine in these two items simply wash out the Vitamin C in your body and no matter how much you put back in with supplements it is a losing battle if you continue to wash it out. That is why I made it a point to tell her that if she really wanted help she would have to help herself first by giving up these two items.

As we applied pressure massage to the response area for the shoulder as shown in Chart 2, the pain began to lessen. The relief was ample proof that help was available.

Two weeks later she was back for another treatment. She had made her choice, cigarettes and coffee had to go. She quit "cold turkey" and was really having withdrawal problems. This along with the Bursitis was about all she could take so we started an intensive program of pressure massage for her pain. In addition to applying Pointed Pressure Massage to the response area on her foot for her shoulder, I instructed her to place rubber bands on her right hand at the first joint on each finger once daily and on the toes of her right foot once daily.

To help her "unwind" just at bedtime she became adept at massaging the response area for general relaxation as shown in Chart 2A. She was free of her problems in eight weeks and could not thank me enough for encouraging her to quit smoking and drinking coffee besides the relief from the shoulder problem of Bursitis.

ARTHRITIS NEED NOT CRIPPLE YOU

Another very common disorder of the joints is Arthritis. This is an inflammation of the joints and is one of the most common and painful abnormalities of the articular system. About fifty varieties are known but the most common are Rheumatoid and Degenerative Arthritis. In Rheumatoid Arthritis there is a general involvement of the connective tissue. It enlarges the tissues and cartilage and stiffens the joint.

Because joints are subject to a great deal of wear and tear after many years of use, degenerative changes set in. Usually this occurs after the age of 45. The weight-bearing joints of the lower extremities and spine are particularly subject to wear and tear and therefore show these degenerative changes. There is a softening of the cartilage, a separation of fibers and eventually actual degeneration of the cartilage.

PRESSURE MASSAGE AWAY THOSE PAINS

Both of these types of Arthritis need never cause you pain and suffering. Your diet is important here because you need an addition of all the Vitamins (A, B, C, D, E) and the trace minerals. Pressure massage can then clear the way to healthy joints.

The Endocrine glands are very closely connected with many problems of dysfunction in the body. If there is a disorder in the body, chances are one or more of the Endocrine glands are involved in some way. This is truly the case with Arthritis. By massaging the response areas for all the Endocrine glands (Thymus, Pineal Thyroid, Parathyroid, Adrenals, Pituitary) as shown in Figures 2A and 2B over a period of a few weeks at least twice weekly, you will be able to straighten out your feet and toes, fingers, elbows and knees. At first you may need someone to apply pressure massage for you until your feet and fingers begin to straighten out. Then you will be able to keep those joints healthy by periodically applying pressure massage yourself. The relief will be unbelievable especially if you think you have tried everything already. Remember, you do not massage the aching joint. You could massage the joint for years and while it won't harm you it is very unlikely that it would do much good. What will give you almost unbelievable results is applying Pointed Pressure Massage to those response areas for the Endocrine glands and the specific problem joints.

When you begin to massage the response area for the Endocrine glands you should start with the Pituitary. While you are directing the massage to the big toe for the Pituitary, you will also be overlapping the response area for the Pineal gland which is just above the Pituitary. Care must be exercised in the first two treatments in any longstanding ailment. The massage must be applied with only moderate pressure and for only a short period of time. Usually this should be about two or three minutes. This allows time for the toxins and poisons which have been accumulated over a period of weeks or months to be eliminated without overloading the kidneys. After the initial removal of these poisons you may increase the pressure applied and the length of time to the full 9 minutes. At this point the massage pressure must be the maximum you can continually apply with your thumb. Don't be afraid to really bear down even though it may hurt a bit. After 9 minutes the sharpness of the response will be somewhat dimmed, however the tenderness will remain as long as the problem or pain continues to bother you. Several weeks of pressure massage may be required to restore normal conditions especially where the glands are out of balance.

Next examine the response area for the Thyroid and repeat the above massage if there is tenderness there. If tenderness persists after massaging the response area for the Thyroid for a period of 8 weeks you may find that you are not getting enough iodine in your diet and may wish to check with your doctor.

Finally, you will massage the response area for the Pancreas and the Adrenal glands as they will most certainly be out of balance in all cases of aching joints. Very often a sugar imbalance exists because of a high intake of starches and sugars and this has either overworked or impaired the insulin machinery to a point that extensive pressure massage is required to restore balance.

You should massage the response area for the Pancreas every other day until the tenderness no longer exists. While you are massaging the response area for the Pancreas you will be taking care of the adrenals since the two areas are almost on top of each other directly in the middle of the bottom of the foot.

A common problem associated with the adrenals is discussed at length in Chapter 10.

You should realize that there are other organs which have response areas which are also in this immediate area. While you are helping one you will be helping several others such as the stomach and salivary glands. You must study the charts carefully to determine the response area for the particular joint which may be bothering you. Two of the most common joint problems to be discussed are the knee and the elbow.

A CASE OF TENNIS ELBOW

I recall one man who came to me with arthritis of the elbow. Mr. R. developed a very painful, disabling condition in his right arm. The elbow became so sore it was almost impossible to bend the arm. Prior to this development of a tennis elbow he had a very strong grip in his hand but gradually he lost most of this grip and could only use his arm for very light tasks. He was unwilling to settle for a temporary relief of pain from aspirin and a lifetime of disablement of the arm. He came to me hoping for some immediate relief and an eventual return of a normal arm.

I began to massage the response area for the elbow on his back as shown in Chart 3. This response area is also for the hand and arm and is therefore very important for any arm problems. As you can see by the figure, this is a response area that you will have to have someone massage for you or you will have to find a mechanical means of doing it yourself. Such a mechanical aid is described in Chapter 3. Another easy way to do this is to drive a nail in a door jamb at just the right height so that the head is exposed about an inch. You can then lean your back against it in such a manner that the nail is pressing on the response area. A similar arrangement is to drill a hole in a board and force a lead pencil in it about half an inch with the metal and eraser remaining exposed. This may be placed in back of you while sitting in a chair to apply pressure massage to the response area for the elbow. It is also useful for problems where the response areas are on the bottom of the feet since you can lay it on the floor and put your foot on it while resting in a chair.

The pain began to leave in a period of four weeks. By continuing this massage every three days, complete relief was had in only ten weeks. Mr. R. began his normal use of his right arm and has not suffered from it since.

Compare this ten weeks of treatment with the years of misery many, many people resign themselves to because they do not know that there is relief for their misery.

A TRICK KNEE CASE

Mr. D. had been interested in athletics while in high school and was able to compete in most of the sports at his school, including football and basketball. He was occasionally bruised in these games but never considered any injury severe. In his third year he began to notice a pain in his left knee. The usual spills always seemed to affect the left knee worse than anywhere else. By the end of the third year he was having so much pain that he had already given up football and was reducing his activity in the other sports. The treatments he was getting were not improving the condition so he was obliged to give up sports entirely for his senior year. When he came to me he had been out of sports for two years and was having trouble walking to and from classes in college. We began Pointed Pressure Massage on the response areas for the knee which are shown in Chart 2B. This area is located on the bottom of your foot near the heel and to the outside of the foot. The area was very tender which made it easy for him to locate on his foot. He lived over forty miles from my office so it was difficult for him to come to my office on a regular basis. I gave him instructions and demonstrated the ways to get the most benefit from pressure massage. He quickly mastered the technique and was able to do the massage himself at home.

At the end of three months he was relieved of most of the discomfort and had returned to near normal use of the leg. The next year saw him back in sports, able to enjoy playing without pain or problems from his trick knee. Twenty years later he runs, golfs and plays tennis without a trace of the problem which was gradually turning him into a cripple during high school.

RHEUMATIC FEVER — SIDE EFFECTS — JOINT PROBLEMS

Another problem that involves the joints is that of Rheumatic Fever. This disease is characterized by inflammation of the connective tissues around the joints. It begins abruptly with an intense inflammatory reaction of the joints and tends to subside after a brief period. When the disease subsides, the patient usually does not show any residual functional damage to the articular system, but frequently there is permanent damage to the heart valves which manifests itself later in life as rheumatic heart disease. Here again we see a connection between the systems. The articular system is the first sight of the problem which next affects the circulatory system. All of this is due to a misbalance or malfunctioning in the Endocrine glandular system. By applying pressure massage on all the glands, particularly the Pituitary, Thyroid, Adrenals and Gonads as shown in Charts 2A and 2B, you can help the system to function properly and eliminate the inflammation that begins in the joints and ends in the heart.

A CASE OF RHEUMATIC FEVER

Mr. A. was always having colds and sore throats. His parents finally decided that his tonsils were the problem and had them removed. Several weeks later the sore throats returned and became more severe as the months passed. Finally he came down with a fever and was bedridden with swollen joints. When he was told he had Rheumatic fever and would be confined to a bed for six months to a year, his parents asked me to give him an examination.

We found the response areas for the throat and the entire Endocrine glandular system very tender. A check for developing heart trouble was negative. This indicated that there was still time to prevent the normal progression of the disease from damaging the heart. We immediately placed him on a saturated Vitamin C program and proceeded to apply Pointed Pressure Massage to the response areas for the throat as shown in Chart 5. By the end of the week we had eliminated the sore throat and the fever. A weekly program of pressure massage to the response areas for the Endocrine glands, Charts 2A and 2B, for three months brought complete relief from the swollen aching joints.

A further check determined that his kidneys were malfunctioning. For some reason he was losing the use of his Vitamin C intake. Massaging the response area for the kidneys in the middle of his foot as shown also in Chart 3 restored normal function to the kidneys. With a continuing program of increasing his intake of Vitamin C and Pointed Pressure Massage he was spared the usual heart problems from this devastating disease.

ARTHRITIS

Mrs. J. began having trouble with her knees when she was 56 years old — four years earlier than when her mother's trouble began. At first she assumed that it was hereditary and nothing could be done for it because her mother had tried everything she could find for it. As the pain increased she began looking for some relief. After trying all of the home remedies available with only partial, temporary relief she came to me to see what "nature had to offer."

TREATMENT:

Pointed Pressure Therapy on the bottom of the foot at the response areas for the knee as shown on Charts 2A and 2B. Thumb pressure for nine minutes on each foot twice weekly for fourteen weeks brought partial relief at each treatment but general relief began to become noticeable during the tenth week. At this point, the improvement was dramatic and complete relief came during the 13th and 14th week when regular treatments were suspended.

There has been no return of the problem and she is in perfect health seven years later. Her mother suffered crippling arthritis in the knees, hips and hands for 30 years. She is confident she can avoid this.

TRICK KNEE

John L. began having problems with his knee which caused him to give up sports in his first year of college. He had been injured only slightly the year before and really couldn't explain why his knee was bothering him. The pain was so severe that he had to limp to walk and tried to stay off his feet as much as possible.

TREATMENT:

Pointed Pressure Therapy to the response area located on the bottom of the foot as shown on Charts 2A and 2B. This is the area which you can give considerable pressure by stepping on a marble and allows you to treat yourself. My treatments were supplemented by his self help efforts at home which actually shortened the length of time required for recovery. We have found that it usually takes about 10 to 20 per cent of the time that the problem has existed to get out of the problem when given proper treatment. In this case he had actually had the problem for over a year and a half but actually didn't come to recognize it until about ten months before he sought help.

LENGTH OF TREATMENT:

Formal treatments lasted for only four weeks. He was so enthused with the possibility of recovery that he worked on his foot regularly and actually did most of the work himself.

Complete recovery allowed him to go back to sports in his second year. After college he began coaching and ten years later he has had no reoccurrence.

RHEUMATIC FEVER

Ms. J. had her tonsils and adenoids removed at the age of eight years. This was during a period of time when the "fad" was to have your tonsils removed at the first sign of sore throat. Months later she realized that this did not stop the sore throats. These became more frequent and severe finally sending her to bed for many months, probably a year.

TREATMENT:

Pointed Pressure Therapy to the response area for the throat and Endocrine glands as shown on Charts 2A and 2B.

LENGTH OF TREATMENT:

As a young doctor, three months of treatment seemed too long for the results we were getting. Consulting another Naturopath, I was reminded even though she was taking three times the MDR of Vitamin C she could have poor utilization of this important vitamin and might require larger quantities. One month after placing her on a saturated vitamin C supplement her recovery was almost complete. While we would have eventually completed her recovery with pressure therapy, any infection related problem yields faster with the help of large amounts of vitamin C. Her recovery, while slow, left her in excellent health — no heart damage. After 20 years she has had no problems.

chapter 5

Helping Your Heart
With Pressure Therapy

The circulatory system consists of the heart, the blood vessels and the blood. The heart acts as a pump which forces the blood through the blood vessels to the various tissues and organs of the body. The walls of the heart are primarily involuntary muscles. In an average adult the heart beats about eighty times a minute. Of course when a person is exercising or excited the heart rate or pulse increases. It also decreases during sleep. It is hard to imagine that a piece of muscle about the size of an adult's fist can do all that the heart does for years without any rest except for the fraction of a second between beats. It is truly an amazing organ.

The heart can be overworked and literally poisoned by overweight, too much salt, coffee and tobacco. As a result the heart will be weakened and will not function properly. Often a heart attack is the final price for mistreating it. To be healthy you must eliminate the above vices. You should apply pressure massage religiously on the response areas for the heart. Look closely at Chart 5. You see the response area for the heart is located just a little more than an inch inside of the left foot. Comparing this with Chart 2 you will note that it is between the thyroid and the stomach as it should be, corresponding with its position in the body. Another important response area for the heart is found on the arm as shown in Chart 5. Use the response area that is most convenient for you to help your own heart. It is very good practice to alternate pressure massage over all the response areas for an organ each time you massage.

If you have already had a heart attack, Pointed Pressure Massage for nine minutes a day every third day will refurbish the heart and help prevent another attack. Also addition of Vitamin E will give the heart a big boost.

HEART ATTACK DUE TO A CRASH DIET

I had a young lady of 20 years brought to my office by her husband. She had already had one heart attack. Being at one time a very heavy lady she had attempted a crash diet by taking reducing pills. She went from 180 pounds to 110 pounds and after this she had her first attack. She survived the attack but was on the verge of a nervous breakdown and exhibited the symptoms of another heart attack in the making. She had pains going up from the heart area to her shoulders and down her arms. It was at this time her husband rushed her to my office for help.

I immediately began pressure massage on the response areas for the heart on the foot and on the arm shown in Chart 5.

After nine minutes of treatment the pain was gone and she began to relax. With continous treatment over a period of three months she was returned to good health. She now is the busy mother of two lovely children.

SUBTLE DIZZINESS MAY BE A WARNING OF HEART TROUBLE

Mr. R. began having pains in his chest which were at first not severe and were ignored as being only a digestive upset. Two weeks later he had another attack of what he thought was indigestion but this time the pain did not leave quickly and he became suspicious of heart problems and decided to have a check-up. He had been overweight and was frequently bothered by a little "dizzy spell" as he called it.

I recognized at once the classical symptoms of impending heart trouble and began applying Pointed Pressure Massage to the heart response area on the left foot. This area was as "sore as a boil" allowing only moderate massage pressure for the first few treatments.

Next we began massaging the response area for general relaxation and for the tight muscles on the back of the neck since tension is generally associated with heart troubles. A gradual weight loss program was begun during the three months' period of pressure massage treatment. This helped him regain a strong healthy heart, thereby avoiding what was sure disaster a few months earlier.

As you can see by these two case histories, overweight is the number one cause of many heart attacks. It is important to loose weight slowly and carefully and then to keep those extra pounds off. If you watch your weight along with tobacco, alcohol and coffee and apply pressure massage to the response areas for the heart you can be assured of a healthy heart and never have to worry about the big killer — heart attack.

Dizziness, as already stated is often associated with heart trouble, problems with blood pressure as well as disorders with blood vessels. By using Pointed Pressure Massage on the response area for circulation on the ear as shown in Chart 4, the blood pressure can be leveled out and the problem of dizziness can be solved.

BLOOD VESSELS

There are three kinds of blood vessels: Arteries, Veins, and Capillaries. Arteries are vessels taking blood away from the heart, veins are the vessels returning the blood to the heart, and capillaries are minute vessels connecting the smallest arteries and veins. They form a network in nearly all parts of the body.

The arteries can become constricted and the vessels become smaller in diameter. When this happens it is harder for the blood to circulate through them and the blood pressure is raised. This is a dangerous condition. Pressure massage on the response areas for the arteries as shown in Chart 6 on the top of the foot, to the outside about two inches just above the tip of the third toe, will open the arteries up and keep them open. High blood pressure will therefore be less of a problem or it will be eliminated completely.

VARICOSE VEINS

Many people, especially women suffer with varicose veins. These are dilations of the superficial veins and usually occur in the legs. The dilation is a result of increased pressure within the veins which occurs if you stand long periods of time or wear clothes that restrict the blood supply. Pregnancy and obesity hasten their development.

By using pressure massage you can do a lot to eliminate varicose veins, especially before they get started. You must of course make sure your clothes are not too tight and that you move your legs periodically if you must stand for a long time. Pressure massage on the response area for circulation on the ear as shown in Chart 4 will help circulation in the legs and thus reduce or eliminate the occurrence of varicose veins.

VARICOSE VEINS HELPED

Mrs. B. began to see the veins in her legs become more prominent as time passed. She also became aware of the beginning of hemorrhoids. Although she saw no connection she was disturbed enough to seek help mainly because she feared disfiguration of her legs or surgery.

She had already begun to add Vitamins E and C to her "new" improved diet and was ready to take the necessary steps to help solve the problem. This was a welcome departure from the average person who wants his health but hangs on to his vices.

We found the response areas for circulation on the legs and face very sensitive and began to apply Pointed Pressure Massage to these areas. Treatment continued for six months at which time the circulation had returned to normal and the veins were only noticeable on close inspection.

If you are beginning to see this impairment of the circulation developing I would urge you to adopt the same program for diet and pressure massage. You must realize that this is a program that takes several months so don't be discouraged if it doesn't clear up in a few days. Continue pressure massage twice weekly until the problem is gone. After you have conquered the problem here are a few don'ts you must know if you are to keep your circulation system in good shape.

1. Don't stand in one position on a hard surface for any length of time.

2. Don't sit with your legs crossed or in a position which slows the circulation.
3. Don't eat foods which have been robbed of Vitamins E or C.
4. Don't be afraid of proper amounts of exercise, preferably walking.

THE BLOOD

Blood vessels form a closed system of tubes for taking blood to various parts of the body and returning it to the heart. The blood is composed of plasma and three main cell types. Red cells, the first type, carry the oxygen throughout the body. If there is a deficiency of red blood cells or the hemoglobin within these cells, anemia develops. Hemoglobin is composed of an iron compound and a deficiency of iron in the system tends to make you anemic. One very obvious symptom is paleness. Pressure massage plus the addition of iron to the system can eliminate this problem. By massaging the response area for blood circulation on the ear you can begin to solve the problem. Anemia is related to problems in the pancreas and spleen so pressure massage on the response areas for these organs helps the blood to become and keep rich in those elements it needs to have the proper chemical balance.

The white blood cells, the second main type of cells, are the soldiers of the body defending it against invasion by disease germs. The number of these vary according to your health but an abnormal increase in the white blood cells leads to leukemia.

The third general type of cells are the platelets which are important in the clotting process. Without the proper number of these, hemophilia results. This is where a person bleeds and bleeds because the blood won't clot properly. Pressure massage on the response area for blood on the leg as shown in Chart 4 helps to restore the proper chemical balance to the blood also.

The functions of the blood are: to carry oxygen to the

different tissues and bring back carbon dioxide, to carry digested food from the digestive tract to the tissues, to remove waste products and carry them to the excretory organs, to control the water content of the body and to regulate the body temperature. So you can see that the blood links all the systems together and is vital in the proper functioning of all of them alone as well as together.

In the average person there is between five and six quarts of blood. The cells are constantly dying and being replaced. General pressure massage of the response area for the blood will insure that these newly formed cells are of the proper composition. Also your diet will play a large role in this proper composition.

When you think of problems with blood you usually think of its circulation or pressure. Improper circulation can complicate all the systems of the body and problems arise everywhere. Since it is very simple and easy to improve your circulation by applying Pointed Pressure Massage to the response area for circulation on the ear, no one should suffer from improper circulation. The same is true for irregular blood pressure. While it is true that low blood pressure is not as serious as high blood pressure it is best to keep our pressure in the norm.

High blood pressure is very common in our society. Indications of it are dizziness as already stated and pains in the back of the head. It commonly leads to strokes and paralysis. Too much salt in the diet often is the culprit for causing high blood pressure. This must be eliminated. After it is eliminated pressure massage can keep your blood pressure within the safe and healthy range. Use pressure massage on the response area for the back of the neck on the outside of the foot as shown in Chart 2B.

CASE OF HIGH BLOOD PRESSURE

I treated Mr. S. T. for constipation, as will be described in Chapter 9. Five years after his treatment for constipation had given him a reprieve on life, Mr. S. T. returned to my office. I gave him an examination and discovered he had high blood pressure. I massaged the response area for circulation on the ear and instructed him to drink a glass of fresh raw fruit juice diluted 50% with water, morning and night along with applying pressure massage for nine minutes every third day to the response areas I had shown him. He followed my advice for a few weeks and began to feel well again. Then he did as many people do when they begin to feel good, he quit drinking the fruit juice and massaging the response areas. He felt great so why should he continue taking his "medicine"? He continued to feel good for quite some time until two years later he had a slight stroke and I was called to his home.

I immediately treated him to lower the pressure by massaging the response areas for the spine along the inside edge of the feet as shown in Charts 2A, 2B and the area for circulation on the ear. In a short time, the pressure was lowered and I instructed him again on where to massage to control his pressure and about the fruit juice. I explained the need for periodic examinations and subsequent pressure massage when the response areas are tender. These areas should be checked and massaged periodically even though you feel okay. Ten years later with this pressure massage treatment and fruit juice he is in excellent health despite his seventy plus years.

PARALYSIS DUE TO HIGH BLOOD PRESSURE

Dr. S. L. had been overweight for over 20 years. His position as administrator and teacher kept him sitting behind a desk every day for years. His hobbies and outside activities were such that he had no physical exercise on the weekends. Without realizing it he had been edging his blood pressure up to a point where he was in danger of real problems such as heart attacks and strokes. A sudden upheaval in the school program adversely affected his work causing him to resign.

The emotional upset was too much for Dr. S. L.'s already weakened cardio-vascular system. A blood vessel broke in the brain area controlling his left arm and leg. He became partially paralyzed in the face and had temporary speech problems.

Massaging the response areas for circulation and paralysis on the face as shown in Chart 4 significantly lowered the blood pressure and began restoring the normal nerve supply. The ruptured blood vessel repaired quickly and as the blood clot dissolved the blockage of the nerve supply was removed so normal movement could be restored. With Pointed Pressure Massage twice weekly for seven months all effects of the stroke disappeared except a very slight area of paralysis on the face. He has become adept at applying pressure massage to the response areas for the heart and circulation and has thus successfully kept from further problems in this vital area.

You two can become adept in treating any problem similar to Dr. S. L.'s once you learn where the response areas are and begin to apply pressure massage. Just think of how this treatment can work for you as it has for many others.

EXTREME NERVOUS EXHAUSTION AND HIGH BLOOD PRESSURE

There are many people who are on the verge of total collapse who are just not aware of how precarious their situation really is.

Your problem may be similar to Mr. B.'s when he came for help. He was "all nerved up." There was an increasing tension in the back of his neck and across his shoulders. He had had a headache for several days which the usual aspirin would not get rid of for him.

I found the area under the small toe on the bottom of the foot as shown in Charts 2A and 2B very tender. Also the area just under the big toe on the side of the foot at the end of the arch was tender, indicating misalignment of a vertebrae in the neck and shoulder area. Nine minutes of pressure massage on these areas twice daily for two weeks corrected his problems.

Do you feel "all nerved up"? Is there an increasing tension across the back of the shoulders and neck area? Have you had a headache for several days which the usual aspirin, etc. will not stop? If you have any of these symptoms or feel dizzy at times you should become sufficiently alarmed to look for the cause immediately. Even if you cannot take your own blood pressure or get it taken right away, there are several things you can do with Pointed Pressure Massage which will restore balance to your system.

First of all you should begin Pointed Pressure Massage on the bottom of the foot just under the base of the little toe. This area will be very tender until the blood pressure returns to normal. It must be massaged with a penetrating rolling motion for at least nine minutes twice daily until things are back to normal.

Secondly, you will find the area under the big toe on the side of the foot to be tender. (Chart 2A and 2B.) This is because there is nearly always a vertebrae in the neck area slightly misaligned when great tension exists in the neck and shoulder area. You will need to apply pressure massage to this area until the vertebrae are realigned. Generally twice daily for nine minutes will be sufficient but you should continue the massage as long as the tension in the shoulder area remains. Treatment can sometimes be stopped in two or three days but sometimes it lasts for several weeks depending on the severity of the problem and on the quality of the pressure massage. For speedy recovery you will have to apply the massage with a vengeance. My motto is "Make it hurt." Remember this is just the opposite of general back rubbing which is meant to be soothing as it is applied. Pointed Pressure Massage is a local, deep penetrating massage.

DROPSY

Heart disease, kidney disease and problems in the liver all contribute to this disorder. It is condition where there is an accumulation of water in the tissues and cavities. Too much sodium and therefore too much salt is the main factor in this disorder. The potassium-sodium balance is upset. A substitution of potassium salts for sodium salts will help and Pointed Pressure Massage will do the rest. Massage the response areas for the heart, kidneys and liver. These areas are shown in Charts 2A and 2B. The heart, as you can see, is only on the left foot. The kidneys are on both and the liver is on the right foot. This corresponds with their position in the body.

A DIAGNOSIS OF LEUKEMIA

Mr. M. suddenly became so weak he had to quit his work and retire. Becoming increasingly weak, he finally sought help. The diagnosis of leukemia shocked him and his family to the point of desperation. His circulatory system was in deep trouble. The pancreas and spleen were atrophied to the point of almost complete failure. We began pressure massage to the response areas to the circulatory system on the face, arm and legs. Next we massaged the areas for the spleen, liver and pancreas. The first four weeks he ate nothing but grapes and took a megavitamin supplement which included Vitamins C and E. This allowed his system to get rid of the toxins and poisons he had accumulated while we were applying pressure massage to his weakened cardio-vascular system. Months later he was feeling normal again, no more transfusions and no more aching legs.

This near tragedy can be averted if you recognize what is happening to you soon enough. If you suddenly loose your normal color, become weak, have bad cramps and aching legs you should begin to apply pressure massage to the response areas for circulation and for the pancreas and spleen. Keep your potassium level high and make sure you are not low in Vitamin C and E.

HEART ATTACK

Mrs. P. was 34 when she realized she was just plain fat and that she should be reducing. Her crash diet was the wrong thing to do. She had been given a few warnings that her heart was rebelling, but she ignored them. When she was brought to my office she was having a "bad seige" similar to the one she had a few days earlier. She thought the pains had something to do with her heart but couldn't believe it was a heart attack.

TREATMENT:

Pointed Pressure Therapy on the left foot as shown on Chart 2B. Rubber bands on the right and left hand and on the right and left foot for nine minutes.

LENGTH OF TREATMENT:

The initial treatment lasted one hour and a half applying the pressure nine minutes and then rubber bands for nine minutes alternately. When the muscles had relaxed sufficiently for her to return home we gave her instructions to apply this therapy once again before bed time, and to return the following morning. We continued treatment every other day for four weeks and advised her to abandon her crash diet in favor of a slow reduction in weight while taking vitamins and minerals. During the next year she lost the weight safely and regained a healthy heart which has maintained its vitality for the past twenty years.

A WORD OF CAUTION:

Any signs of heart attack should be immediately brought to the attention of your doctor, since time is an important factor in prevention and treatment. In the previous case history, my examination revealed no major cause for alarm. She had been fortunate to have had only a minor attack which did not require hospitalization. In most cases this therapy is best for prevention and or treatment before an actual heart attack has been experienced but many have regained a healthy heart by using this therapy even following a severe attack.

HIGH BLOOD PRESSURE

Mr. B. was not aware that he had high blood pressure. His headaches and nervousness were what he thought was part of getting past 40. One day he was attempting to loosen a bolt on a machine and was straining more than he realized. Suddenly he felt a sting in his left eye. He thought something had blown in it so he came to my office to have it removed. Close examination revealed a large area which was blood shot but nothing had blown in the eye. His blood pressure was 145/95 — high enough for any blood vessel to break. He was lucky. This could have been a blood vessel in the brain and that could have caused paralysis or even death.

TREATMENT:

Pointed Pressure Therapy applied to the response area for the 7th cervical and 1st and 2nd thoracic vertebrae as shown on Charts 2A and 2B. A reducing diet to trim off 40 lbs. of excess weight and to cut out salt.

LENGTH OF TREATMENT:

Three months of treatment to correct the spinal problems and another four months to control the weight problem.

I have never had a case of High Blood pressure in which there
were no problems in the neck area. I believe the vertebrae are
pulled out of place by tension in the shoulder area. This in turn
is usually accompanied by some dietary deficiency, usually
the B vitamins and or some unpleasant or stress condition
which causes worry. With the application of Pointed Pressure Therapy we can break the vicious cycle of tension-
caused high blood pressure. Many strokes could be avoided
by this easy way to lower dangerous blood pressure levels.

chapter 6

How To Treat
Stomach Problems

The digestive system consists of the mouth and its associated structures, the pharynx, the esophagus, the stomach, the small intestine, the liver, the gall bladder and pancreas, the large intestine, the rectum, and the anus. It is concerned with the intake and digestion of food so that it can be utilized by the body. The system also stores excess food and eliminates the solid waste products of digestion.

Years of improper living habits, particularly poor eating can eventually take its toll on the digestive system. We eat too much food which has been processed in a manner that either removes essential elements from it or adds unwanted items such as preservatives.

Cooking destroys the enzymes so we recommend eating fresh, raw foods as much as possible. Most of our fruits and vegetables are sprayed with insecticides which have a oily base and so must be thoroughly cleaned by using soap and water solutions. There are some commercial cleaning agents for this purpose but care must be taken in rinsing so that whatever the solution used, it is removed entirely.

RELIEF FROM ITCHING ANUS

There are many problems that can develop within the organs of the digestive system. For example in the anal area, itching may cause a lot of discomfort if not treated. This is often caused by an allergy to foodstuffs or to the wood products in toilet paper. By using Pointed Pressure Massage on the response area to the anus, this irritation can be relieved in a short time.

Seat yourself in a comfortable position so you can hold your foot and apply pressure with your thumb on the response area to the anus on the bottom of your foot as shown in Chart 2B.

COLITIS DISAPPEARS

Another problem occurs when the colon is inflamed (colitis). This also can be relieved by simply massaging the response areas for the colon as shown in Chart 2B.

YOU CAN RESTORE YOUR LIVER

The liver, which is the largest organ in the body, has many functions. It filters blood from the digestive tract and produces bile to digest fats. Some of the problems in the liver include atrophy, accumulation of excess poisons, jaundice, and schlerosis due to drinking alcoholic beverages. In Chart 2A you will find the response area for the liver. It is approximately in the center of the foot but to the outside and covers an area about the size of a quarter. When applying pressure massage to this area, you should massage thoroughly the entire area every other day until the tenderness is gone.

GALL STONES DISSOLVED
BY PRESSURE MASSAGE

Within this area is the response area for the gall bladder also. The gall bladder is on the underside of the right lobe of the liver. It is a sac where the bile formed by the liver is temporarily stored. A common problem arising within the gall bladder or bile ducts is that of gall stones. This is a deposit of calcium in the shape of small stones. They are usually due to a poor diet and a deficiency of vitamins. By applying pressure massage on the response area for the gall bladder within the response area of the liver as shown also in Chart 2A, once a week for about twenty weeks, these painful stones can be dissolved. They must be broken up and dissolved slowly so as not to cause a blockage. Therefore the treatment must be over a period of about twenty weeks.

APPENDIX AND ILEO-CECAL VALVE

The entrance from the small intestine is called the ileocecal valve. When this entrance is restricted or inflamed (ileitis) you are overcome with acute pain. This pain is often confused with the pain in appendicitis, which is the restriction, inflammation and swelling of the entrance to the appendix. If you study Chart 2A, you will see that the response area for these two problems are very close together so pressure massage in this area will relieve any blockage in this region, dilate the appendix, and thus relieve pressure in it. If the appendix is ruptured, surgical intervention will be necessary immediately.

A CASE OF APPENDICITIS RELIEVED

I have had many patients with acute appendicitis come to me but the one that is most clear in my mind is the case of my daughter. One day she came home from college with a pain in the area of the appendix. She told me she felt the pain earlier that day but that it was mild and she thought it was just gas and would go away. As the day went on, it didn't go away and by the time I arrived home she was bent over in pain. I immediately began to massage the response area for the appendix on the bottom of the foot about three inches from the heel and a half inch from the outside of the foot as shown in Chart 2A. The area was very tender and I continued pressure massage for about an hour until she could straighten up again and the pain was relieved. The next day the area on the bottom of the foot was so sore she could hardly walk on it but shortly the tenderness was gone and the pain in the area of the appendix was completely removed and has never reappeared.

MALABSORPTION CAN ROB YOUR BODY OF VITAL NUTRIENTS

A common problem in the intestinal area of the digestive tract is that of malabsorption. This is the failure of the intestinal tract to absorb nutrients properly from digested food and is caused by toxins within the system. By applying pressure massage to the response areas of the intestines as shown in Chart 4 these toxins may be eliminated and absorption will become normal again.

Hold your foot so that you can apply pressure to the entire middle section of the foot. Apply deep penetrating massage to the entire area, dwelling particularly on any extra tender spots. Each and every tender response area should receive a full nine minutes of pressure massage twice a week.

THE STOMACH

The stomach is a sac-like organ which serves mainly as a storage center for food prior to its passage into the small intestine. It does permit some digestion of food within it even though this is not its main function. The normal capacity of an adult stomach is about 1-1/2 quarts. Three to four hours are usually required for a meal to pass through an adult stomach. Four common problems associated with the stomach are that of dyspepsia, ulceration, colic and gas.

DYSPEPSIA AND COLIC

Dyspepsia is imperfect digestion due to a failure of the system to produce the proper digestive juices and enzymes and an improper diet. It is often accompanied by nausea and vomiting. Colic is also indigestion. It is associated with gas and abdominal pain. For both dyspepsia and colic you can apply pressure massage on the response areas to the stomach for lasting relief. As shown in Charts 2A, 2B, the response area for the stomach is on the inside of both feet about a half inch above the middle of the foot. It should be massaged in a rolling manner for nine minutes every third day.

GAS

If gas is a problem, pressure massage on the front of the leg as shown in Chart 3, will relieve it after a few minutes.

How many times have you had a gas or indigestion problem at a place or time when an antacid tablet was not available? It is at times like this that you can rid yourself of the gas with pressure massage.

As we grow older the digestion of our food becomes less complete. This natural slow down is accompanied by excess gas and accompanying discomfort. For many people adding enzymes can help this problem but the real solution can be found in Pointed Pressure Massage. A healthy digestive tract can provide proper digestive juices and enzymes needed for complete assimilation of ingested food particles. By massaging the response areas for the stomach and intestines you will be covering the areas for other important organs such as the pancreas. You should continue this pressure massage every other week even after your localized discomfort is gone, for in so doing you will maintain good digestion. This is a most essential element in good health and a way to slow down the aging process.

A CASE HISTORY OF GAS RELIEF

Mr. C. came to me with a pain in his right side which he thought might be his appendix. He had been having these pains frequently for several weeks but they were on the increase in frequency and duration. After having a bowel movement or the expulsion of gas he generally felt better for a while. Since he showed none of the other symptoms of appendicitis, we looked for tenderness all along the intestinal tract. Several areas were sore including both the large intestine and small intestine and the pancreas. His diet, which was heavy in starch and sugar, had overloaded the insulin-producing machinery and this caused imperfect utilization of the starches and sugar resulting in gas formation.

Pointed Pressure Massage to these response areas, brought immediate relief but it took several weeks to restore the balance in the glandular system. A reduction of starches and sugars took the heavy load off the insulin producers while the pressure massage was completing the restorative process. He can now obtain temporary relief from overeating etc. by applying pressure massage to the center of his foot.

ULCERS

The stomach glands secrete acids to soften and breakdown the food. An over secretion of these acids due to a bad diet, deficiency of B and C vitamins, worry, stress and nerves, can cause peptic ulceration. Ulcers, in the stomach or duodenum (the first part of the small intestine), are open lesions in the mucosal wall of these organs. Symptoms of ulceration include loss of weight, fainting, nervousness, dark stools, insomnia and pain in the area of the stomach. Faithful application of Pointed Pressure Massage will relieve the pain of ulcers and over a period of time eliminate them completely.

A CASE OF ULCERS CURED

Mr. L. married at the age of twenty with only one year of college. Lacking a trade he was able to gain employment only as a day laborer at a salary too low to afford him the luxuries he and his wife had known while growing up. He was constantly having problems in meeting his bills and this began to affect his nerves. Before he could sort out his difficulties he became aware of a recurring "pain in the stomach." By the time his third child was born he was fearful he would have to be in the hospital for an operation.

When he asked for help he was unaware of the complications that had brought him to his bad health. His first treatment by Pointed Pressure Massage was aimed primarily at relieving the tension that kept him "tied up in knots" most of the time. We massaged the response area for general relaxation and the response area for the back of the neck as shown in Chart 2A. This unwound him and as a result he was able to have his best night of rest and sleep in many weeks. Then we began a series of treatments massaging the response area for the stomach as shown also in Chart 3. This response area remained sore for

over three months even though we massaged it twice a week for
nine minutes each time. During this period he became acquainted with the response areas for relaxation and would
massage them instead of taking a sleeping pill. He also changed
his diet to fresh raw fruits and vegetables, giving up his fried
foods, pop and bakery goods which he had learned were part
of his problem. Realizing that health was more important than
material things helped him forego buying things compulsively.
His finances were becoming manageable before he was pro-
moted on the job and became the least of his worries after the
promotion. He broke the cycle of worry, bad health and finan-
cial problems in the few months of pressure massage on the
response areas for insomnia, ulcers, and nervous tension.

In the years that followed he has kept his good health by
close attention to good living habits. Nine minutes of Pointed
Pressure Massage for general relaxation occasionally helps him
get to sleep without sleeping pills but there has been no return
of his digestive problems or nervous tension since then.

CONSTIPATION — CURSE
OF MODERN CIVILIZATION

One of the most common problems associated with the
digestive system is that of constipation. It is caused chiefly
by a poor diet but there are many other factors which add to
the problem.

If you are forced to eat your meals at irregular hours,
this can upset the system and thus cause constipation. An
inadequate intake of fluids further complicates the problem
because your system requires a minimal amount of fluid and
without this certain amount, which is different for everyone,
it will not function properly.

In addition to poor diet, another chief cause of constipation is simply that we ignore the call of nature too many
times. We are just too busy, too regimented to take the

necessary time to have a bowel movement at the time of the greatest urge. Working conditions, school pressures or the mere absence of toilet facilities at the proper time cause a postponement which is detrimental to our health.

The first rule then is to correct the diet and the second is to provide a time for a bowel movement when the urge is the greatest.

A LONGSTANDING CASE OF CONSTIPATION CURED WITH PRESSURE MASSAGE

Patients who come to me for help with constipation usually have tried everything they know in the form of laxatives. They usually have been in trouble for long periods of time and have other problems along with or as a result of constipation.

Mr. S. came to my office having been told that he was nearing the end since he was so full of tumors of the rectum that he could not survive an operation. He told me that his condition was so bad that he had to resort to drinking a quart of hot salt water to move his bowels. He was very discouraged and asked if there was anything I could do to help him. I told him to sit down and relax and in a matter of a few minutes he would be able to have a natural bowel movement without drinking the hot salt water. He sat down and I immediately gave him a Pointed Pressure Massage treatment on the response area for constipation on his chin, on the front of it and on the bottom as shown in Chart 4 for nine minutes. I then massaged the response area for constipation on the cheek bones below the ridge at the bottom of the eyes as shown in Chart 4, for another nine minutes. In approximately twenty minutes he was ready to have his first natural bowel movement in six months.

After relieving himself, I discussed with him at length the necessity of revamping his eating and living habits. I continued the Pointed Pressure Massage for several months after this. During this time he learned the rudiments of healthy living and became proficient in massaging the response areas for constipation for himself. His return to health confounded those who thought he had but a short time to live.

AN ACUTE CASE OF CONSTIPATION

A very common beginning of constipation problems is childbirth. Mrs. C. had always been regular prior to her pregnancy. She had been careful to eat a balanced diet and had been accustomed to regular hours for eating. This regularity had been easy for her to maintain because there was no regimentation which kept her from visiting the bathroom whenever the urge came to her. The fact that she did not have to meet a rigid schedule, which most working people follow, left her free to set her own time table.

When pregnancy upset this mode of living, she began relying on an occasional laxative in an attempt to be regular. She believed that normal habits could be resumed after the baby was born. Actually things became worse. She was up at odd hours of the night, ate convenience foods and failed to drink enough fluids. Breast feeding the baby increased the need for fluid intake which she failed to do. By this time she was relying on laxatives most of the time but realized that something needed to be done to break the cycle. She knew something had changed but assumed it was the result of pregnancy.

Her first call for help was prompted by a blockage which her now regular laxative had failed to move. She was frightened because someone had told her that surgery was sometimes necessary in severe cases.

YOU CAN THROW AWAY LAXATIVES FOREVER

After determining the nature of the laxatives she was using and the length of time since the last bowel movement it was evident that a normal movement was possible since the fecal material was not compacted enough to prevent passage.

By applying Pointed Pressure Massage to the response area for constipation on the tip of the coccyx as shown in Chart 4 for nine minutes we relaxed the rectal area. I then applied pressure massage under the chin as shown in Chart 4 for the same length of time. Both response areas were very tender indicating that the constipation was severe even though it was of short duration. A normal bowel movement within a half-hour began her return to regularity. She began to rebuild her earlier good habits and learned to apply the Pointed Pressure Massage to the chin and just below the ridge on the cheek bone below the eyes as shown in Chart 4, to re-establish regular bowel movements. In a period of six weeks she was back to normal and had to apply Pointed Pressure Massage only once in the following year. She was delighted that she no longer had to rely on a laxative for temporary constipation.

HEMORRHOIDS - ANOTHER CURSE OF MODERN CIVILIZATION

Often associated with constipation is modern man's problem of hemorrhoids. This is usually a very painful condition which is brought on by the same regimented life associated with constipation. Refined foods, failure to respond to the natural urge to defecate, not enough fluid intake, make the bowel movement so difficult that the lining of the rectum becomes distended. Repeated straining causes the vertical folds which contain veins to become enlarged. The enlargement of veins is known as hemorrhoids or piles.

SHRINKING HEMORRHOIDS

Most long standing cases of constipation result in complications for the digestive system. Mr. G. began relying on laxatives after he had been having problems with constipation for several years. Forcing evacuation of the bowels had given him internal and external hemorrhoids. He was reluctant to have surgery because his father had died of cancer following surgery for a fistula which had a malignant growth. There was no reason to believe this was true in his case so we began a series of Pointed Pressure Massage treatments aimed at correcting not only the painful hemorrhoids but the constipation which had caused them.

First we began working on the response area for hemorrhoids found in Chart 6 because he was having so much pain especially from the protruding veins which were swollen and sore. The response area, which you can see in Chart 2A, on the back of the heel was very tender and remained that way for several weeks. By massaging this area very thoroughly for nine minutes every other day we were able to gradually reduce the pain and swelling.

DISCARD LAXATIVES

At the same time we were massaging the response area for hemorrhoids we massaged the response area for constipation on the chin and under the cheek bones as shown in Chart 4. In a few weeks he was able to discontinue the laxatives and only occasionally needed an enema. He started a program of diet correction, increased his fluid intake between meals and provided a regular schedule for proper living. Applying Pointed Pressure Massage to all these areas discussed became a regular part of his daily life. One day he would massage the areas on the face for constipation and the next day the areas on the heel for hemorrhoids.

This effort was marked with real success. A year later he was able to vacation for six weeks in his camper on a trip covering over 8,000 miles. This was entirely out of the question twelve months earlier because his hemorrhoids were so painful he could only ride in a car for short distances on necessary errands such as shopping.

CONSTIPATION

Mr. D. had suffered from bleeding piles and severe constipation for fifteen years. Then the pain of elimination became unbearable and he had "made the rounds" before coming to me. Rejecting surgery was not an easy decision because he was able to evacuate the bowels only with the help of strong laxatives and even then with severe pain.

TREATMENT:

Pointed Pressure Therapy on the response area on the chin as shown on Chart 4 for nine minutes, sent him to the bathroom for his first bowel movement, without a laxative for years.

LENGTH OF TREATMENT:

Two treatments per week consisting of nine minutes of pressure on the chin were required for six months. In addition to these treatments, the patient learned to apply the pressure before each bowel movement. Recovery, though slow, was dramatic enough to keep him "working at it." At the end of four months most of the bleeding was gone and the pain was entirely gone. Formal treatments were over in six months. Eleven years later he is in good health — no more problems with constipation.

HEMORRHOIDS

Ms. L. suddenly began having problems with hemorrhoids after the birth of her second boy. Fluid intake was not adequate especially since she was nursing. This caused very hard compacted stools and resulted in painful evacuation.

TREATMENT:

Addition of fluids to her diet seemed to have little effect so I began a series of Pointed Pressure Therapy treatments for constipation and hemorrhoids on the face as shown on Chart 4 and on the foot as shown on Chart 6.

LENGTH OF TREATMENT:

Nine minutes three times weekly for each response area for the total of five weeks.

Recovery was complete in five weeks but most symptoms were gone in three weeks. The stool became soft allowing easy passage and this let the rectal area return to normal.

Condition has remained normal for the past twelve years. What probably would have become a chronic condition was prevented by proper care.

ULCERS

Mr. Jim B. thought he was too young at 22 to have ulcers, but he had them anyway. Milk and crackers every two hours and all other useless "treatments" for ulcers were doing him no good. A friend asked him to see me and find out what I could do for him. When anyone has ulcers or thinks he has them I advise him to take it seriously. Any sign of blood in the stool should be ample warning that something is wrong.

TREATMENT:

Over the years we have concluded that ulceration is a deficiency disease — lack of proper food elements. Fresh raw foods or juices plus vitamin C and E will usually prevent ulcers but once you have them you usually need pressure therapy plus the right foods and vitamins to restore balance to the system.

LENGTH OF TREATMENT:

Pressure therapy to the response area which is affected as shown on Charts 2A and 2B for nine minutes twice weekly for three months restored Jim's health. His zest for raw fresh foods has insured him that it will not return.

ITCHING ANUS

Mr. K. began having puritis anus when he started working in the grain mill and perspiring heavily. He had previously been working at a job where he did little manual labor and therefore perspired moderately. When the itching became unbearable he began trying the usual home remedies and later several prescriptions, none of which helped. The Naturopathic approach to disease assumes there is something missing in the diet or that there is something abnormal in the environment. Nature usually can restore balance to our bodies. When this does not happen, help must be given which will assist the natural, recuperative processes.

When Mr. K. came to me, he had quit his new job and returned to his old job because he thought sweating might be his problem, but this did not help.

TREATMENT:

Pointed Pressure Therapy to the response area for the anus as shown on Charts 2A and 2B.

Most people who have colds frequently or have low grade infections constantly do not get enough of Vitamins A, C and E in their diet. A complete overhaul of his diet was necessary but even that would not have corrected the problem without help.

LENGTH OF TREATMENT:

Itching problems are very difficult to correct and usually take many weeks of pressure therapy but in his case only nine weeks were required because he learned where and how to apply the pressure and cooperated in all aspects of the treatment including his diet revolution.

Today his health is excellent and he has had no more skin problems.

COLITIS

Mrs. C. had constant abdominal pain with alternating diarrhea and constipation. She had a dull, aching pain and feeling of uneasiness and discomfort along the entire large intestine. Sometimes the attacks were severe, lasting several hours and were followed by the passage of stringy, tough mucus. Much of the pain is caused by the efforts of the bowel to rid itself of the mucus which adheres to the bowel. As is often the case with colitis, she was thin, pale, anemic and poorly nourished.

TREATMENT:

Pressure Therapy to the response areas on the foot as shown in Charts 2A and 2B. This requires pressure at several points along the colon and therefore is longer than most treatment periods. Nine minutes at the illeo-cecum response area on Monday; nine minutes at the middle of the ascending colon on Tuesday; nine minutes at the top of the transverse colon on the right foot response area on Wednesday; nine minutes on the left foot transverse colon response area on Thursday; nine minutes on the response area for the descending colon on Friday; nine minutes on the sigmoid colon response area on Saturday and finally nine minutes on the anal response area on Sunday. This treatment must be accompanied with drinking only raw vegetable juices the first week and then eating only raw vegetables one week and raw fruits the next alternately for as much as six weeks. Mrs. C. was free from pain and flatulence by the end of the six week period and has remained free from the problem for twelve years having excellent health at the present time.

CAUTION:

In ulcerative colitis, where there is evidence of blood in the stool, no manipulative treatments should be given until the patient has been on raw cabbage juice for at least a week. This allows time for the mucus to disappear without causing severe pain and bleeding.

APPENDIX

Mrs. H. had frequent attacks of appendicitis which were painful and upsetting but none so bad that she felt she should see someone or have them removed. The frequency was to a point she felt she should now see if something could be done before it got so bad that an operation would be required. While she didn't consider these attacks dangerous, I view any attack of appendicitis as potentially dangerous and would suggest consulting your doctor in any event as a precautionary measure.

TREATMENT:

If the attack can be alleviated within a few minutes by pressure therapy to the response area for the appendix as shown on Chart 2A, it is then possible to rid yourself of the reoccurring problems by applying this pressure for nine minutes every other day for three weeks.

In Mrs. H's case, I felt the attack was severe enough that I began a series of routine lab tests, while applying the pressure therapy, just in case there might be a need for surgery.

Fortunately the attack was quickly relieved by Pointed Pressure Therapy and did not require surgery.

LENGTH OF TREATMENT:

Four weeks of treatments twice weekly cleared up the congestion and she was free of further attacks.

It is my belief that you should keep your appendix if you can keep healthy because it is known to be a germ fighter and is also a blow-off valve for excess pressure.

Her problems have been gone for nine years and today she is in very good health.

ILEO-CECAL VALVE

Mr. P. would have thought he was having frequent attacks of appendicitis had he not known he had his appendix removed twenty years earlier. He wanted to know if it could regrow, many people confuse the two since the pain, location etc. is similiar. In his case, examination revealed a hard lump about the size of a tennis ball at the site of the ileo-cecal valve. It was obvious that the pain was caused by the swelling which was blocking the movement of food through the tract. Tests were inconclusive, so we elected to use pressure therapy.

TREATMENT:

We applied Pointed Pressure Therapy to the response area for the ileo-cecal valve as shown on Chart 2A.

LENGTH OF TREATMENT:

The pain and swelling began to leave after three treatments. In five weeks there was no sign of pain or swelling in the side. What might have ended in an operation for ileitis was avoided.

Many cases of ileitis have been incorrectly diagnosed as appendicitis and operations performed for the wrong thing. President Eisenhower's operation brought to the attention of the American people that there was more than one reason for severe pain in the right side. In his case it had progressed so far that surgical intervention was necessary and quick.

Don't presume on fate — that pain in your side could kill you without proper treatment. With Pointed Pressure Therapy you can avoid serious consequences.

chapter 7

How To Help
Your Kidneys

The urinary system consists of those organs used in excretion. These organs are the kidneys, the ureters, the urinary bladder and the urethra.

The kidneys are located towards the back of the abdomen just above the waistline. They are bean-shaped organs. Within each kidney are about one million little filter systems called the nephrons. This is where the kidneys do their work, filtering 1200 ml of blood every minute. Here 99% of the fluid is reabsorbed. The 1% left goes out of the kidneys and down the ureters, the two tubes which convey urine from the kidneys to the urinary bladder which serves as a reservoir for the urine. It gradually fills and becomes distended which causes an increase in pressure within the bladder. A voluntary control of the brain then results in micturition. Upon micturition, the urine leaves the bladder through the urethra and is thus excreted.

BEDWETTING

Enuresis, an involuntary bedwetting during sleep by a child over three years of age, is a problem which can be helped by Pointed Pressure Massage. It can be caused by many factors including a local irritation of the urinary bladder and urethra, emotional instability, overtiredness, and a bad diet of too much white sugar and white flour products. Pressure massage on the response area for bedwetting on the lower back as shown in Chart 5 for nine minutes every third day will establish the normal voluntary response and eliminate the involuntary bedwetting.

A CASE OF BEDWETTING

Elaine had rarely slept through a night without wetting the bed in her first 10 years of living. Repeated attempts to find the cause had failed. Her parents had tried everything they could find to help her solve the problem. She had tried to abstain from drinking any fluid three hours prior to going to bed with no success. Her medical test revealed nothing which could be contributing to the problem. Repeated examinations found her completely normal and yet the problem persisted.

A lengthy discussion of her problem began to yield some of the underlying reasons for her continuing misfortune. Candy and soda pop were very much a part of her diet. Over many years most of my patients with kidney problems have been those who ate too much starch and sugar and drank too little water. She was a typical case.

The response areas for the kidneys shown in Chart 2B were very tender and remained sensitive for about 8 weeks of treatment. We also found that the endocrine glands were full of problems. The pituitary, thyroid, adrenals and pancreas were not functioning properly. Pointed Pressure Massage on the response areas for these glands quickly restored their normal functioning. Although she still wanted candy she was glad to curtail her eating of it enough to aid her body to function properly. She was no longer afraid to go to a slumber party with her girl friends or to a summer camp. She had learned at a very early age that you cannot abuse your body and keep it healthy.

ANOTHER CASE OF BEDWETTING

Ed N. had resigned himself to a life time of bedwetting when numerous attempts to obtain help had failed to improve his condition. His parents had taken him to specialist after specialist in an attempt to correct his problem. At the age of 18 he started college and, fearful that his problem would be known, requested a single room. He made it through one year without anyone learning his secret but had acquired a girl-friend and wanted to get married.

A fellow classmate of his who had been to me for treatment, Joe D., learned of Ed's problem and suggested that he give it one more try. Joe told Ed that he had also been told his condition was incurable and found out that that was not the case. Joe had been completely cured of arthritis of the knee.

During his first visit I discovered Ed ate candy at a rate that was almost unbelievable. The response areas for the kidneys and the pancreas were exceptionally tender. This indicated that he was overloading the kidneys with sugar and that his insulin-producing machinery was also overworked.

We began a program of Pointed Pressure Massage on the response area for the kidneys and pancreas shown in

Chart 2A. The pancreas response area just below the nose
was so tender at first I thought he might have an abscessed
tooth but realized that was not possible since he had been
wearing dentures for several years.

I explained that the overloading of the kidneys and the
pancreas by his excessive eating of candy would thwart the
treatment. Ed was gaining interest in his health and agreed
to limit his eating of candy to two candy bars a week. When
he did not improve after the first week he was very discouraged but agreed to continue the pressure massage treatments
for two more weeks. During the second week he slept two
nights without wetting the bed, something he had not done
as far back as he could remember. This was too good to be
true! By now he was eagerly mastering the massage technique
hoping to become a "normal boy." The formal treatments
ended in six weeks when he was only "missing" occasionally.
He continued massaging the response areas and in another
3 months he was rid of his problem. When school was out the
end of his second year he got married and has had no problem
since.

RENAL INSUFFICIENCY

Miss B. was always tired even when she had plenty
of rest. When she was overly tired her eyes became puffy
and swollen. Minor pains in the abdomen, swollen ankles and
constant headaches were mute reminders that her kidney
problems were not getting better. When she began having
blurred vision, a sense of urgency sent her looking for help.
She had been told that her kidneys were just not capable of
removing as much waste as she made daily. This was before
the development of the kidney machine so there really wasn't
much that could be offered. A friend suggested Pointed Pressure Massage because she had previously been helped with
this system of therapy.

Candy and starchy foods were part of her problem but she needed a lot of convincing to change her diet. I agreed to give her pressure massage only if she would cut out sweets and starchy foods for a trial period of two months. During that time I felt sure we could correct her problem and show her the road to good health.

We began massaging the response areas for the kidneys and for the endocrine glands as shown in Charts 2A and 2B. Her immediate improvement was a welcome surprise. She quickly learned the places to apply the pressure massage and did such a good job that she only had to return every other week so we could check her progress. At the end of three months she needed no persuasion to keep her diet correction in force. Good health was ample reason for her to eat right.

Once fearful of marriage, she soon forgot her problem and married within the year. Fifteen years later her health was still excellent. Four successful pregnancies had in no way given any indications of her earlier kidney problems.

CONGESTION

Besides problems of bedwetting and renal insufficiency there is the problem of congestion. If there is a problem with the kidneys and the endocrine glands, congestion can be a problem. This can cause backaches, gas, cramps and general aching.

CONGESTION CURED

Many people such as Mrs. C. do not realize the importance of drinking enough fluids. Others drink enough fluids but drink the wrong things. Tea, coffee, alcoholic beverages and soft drinks are injurious to your health. Mrs. C. was a coffee drinker and used so much salt that she was ruining her lower bowels and kidneys. She drank about four cups of coffee a day and that was all the fluid she got except for the fluids in the foods she ate. Her legs and ankles were always swollen and she felt listless. I agreed to treat her provided she cut out all salt from her diet and stop drinking coffee. Reluctantly she agreed and we began applying Pointed Pressure Massage to the response areas for the kidneys and lower intestines. In ten days she was feeling much better in spite of the coffee addiction. For the first time in years she was drinking plain water and determined to continue. When the swelling was gone and she regained her zest for living she was sure it was all worth it.

If you have these problems you are courting real disaster if you don't look for help. Begin to apply Pointed Pressure Massage to the response areas for the kidneys and intestines as shown in Chart 2A, and correct your eating and drinking habits at once. You have everything to gain and nothing to lose except a couple of bad habits.

chapter 8

Revitalize Your Glands With Pointed Pressure Massage

The endocrine glands include the thyroid, the parathyroids, the adrenals, the pancreas, the pituitary, the pineal, the ovaries and the testes. The proper functioning of these glands is vital to a healthy body and treatment of their response areas will prevent trouble from developing in any other part of the body.

THE THYROID

The thyroid is one of the best known of the endocrine glands because it is the one involved in goiters. It is composed of two lobes lying on both sides of the trachea. The gland has one of the best blood supplies of any organ in the body. It is an important gland because its hormone, thyroxin is necessary for normal physical and mental development. It is also important in the retention of water, bone development and the proper functioning of the sex organs. Pressure massage on the response area for the thyroid as shown in Chart 2B will keep the thyroid functioning properly again.

THE PARATHYROIDS

On the back of the thyroid gland, on its surface are the parathyroid glands. The hormone parathormone, secreted by these glands, regulates the calcium ion concentration of the body fluids and is very important in the health of the bones and blood. When there is a deficiency of calcium, the maintenance of equilibrium in the system is impaired. If the parathyroids are not functioning properly, the necessary concentration of calcium will not be maintained. Pressure massage on the response area for the parathyroids as shown just below the metatarsal bone of the big toe in Chart 2A and within the response area of the thyroid, will keep the parathyroids functioning properly.

THE ADRENALS

There are two adrenal glands, one lying above each kidney. Each gland has a cortex or outer portion and a medulla or inner portion. The medulla secretes the hormone adrenalin, and in times of emergency or danger, adrenalin is secreted in greater amounts than usual in order to prepare the body for whatever action is necessary. When this happens many organs and tissues react together. Therefore proper functioning of the adrenal glands is necessary for many of the coordinated body activities.

The cortex of the adrenal gland is necessary for life. Without it death would occur. It secretes the hormone cortin which is involved in the normal use of water, sodium and potassium by the body. It also is important in regulating the use of carbohydrates. These four things must be kept in proper balance in the body. With Pointed Pressure Massage on the adrenal gland as shown in Chart 2A this maintenance can be insured.

THE PANCREAS

The pancreas is important in digestion as well as an important endocrine gland. It is made up of many little islets called the Islets of Langerhans and is located underneath the stomach and just above the kidneys.

COMBATING LOW BLOOD SUGAR AND DIABETES

The pancreatic hormone is insulin, which is necessary for the normal use of sugar and fats. The insulin takes sugar out of the blood stream according to its need. If there is an excess of insulin secreted (hyperinsulinism) then too much sugar is taken out and low blood sugar results. This makes you hungry, weak, sweat a lot, and eventually, if this condition is not corrected, you may go into a coma and die. On the other hand, if there isn't enough insulin secreted (diabetes mellitus) then the blood has too much sugar in it and these symptoms develop: increased thirst, frequent urination, itching, loss of weight, weakness, nausea, headache, vomiting, which may be followed by a deep coma and death. Insulin insufficiency can also lower your resistance to infections.

Both of these harmful problems can be improved and in some cases eliminated by helping the pancreas regulate or improve its production as the case may be. By applying Pointed Pressure Massage to the response areas for the pancreas, particularly the Islets of Langerhans, you can return the function of this organ to a normal condition. If you will look at the chart of the endocrine glands again you will notice that the response area for the pancreas is within that of the stomach. The pancreas is just below the stomach so therefore its response area is correspondingly below that of the stomach. See Charts 2A and 2B.

THE PITUITARY

The pituitary gland, a small organ about the size of a pea, is located in the middle of the head. It is usually called the master gland because it has so many important functions. Many of these functions are mediated through the other endocrine glands. It is divided up into two lobes, an anterior and a posterior one. The anterior lobe secretes 6 different hormones that control many activities and organs of the body. The growth hormone regulates the growth of various organs and parts of the body. The thyrotrophic hormone stimulates the thyroid gland to secrete its hormone thyroxine. The ACTH stimulates the cortex of the adrenal gland to secrete its hormone. The gonadotrophic hormones act on the gonads (ovaries and testes) to stimulate them to secrete their hormones. The lactogenic hormone causes the secretion of milk by the breasts after the birth of a baby.

The posterior lobe secretes pituitrin which acts on the circulatory system, smooth muscles, water absorption by the kidneys, and the metabolism of sugar. It raises the blood pressure, slows down the heart beat and speeds up the rate of breathing. Failure of this lobe to secrete its hormones can affect many systems of the body and cause diabetes insipidus.

GOOD HEALTH FOR YEARS TO COME

As you can see the pituitary gland does indeed control and affect the other glands as well as all the systems in the body. Balance within the endocrine glandular system depends on the pituitary. If you have any problem with this gland, or any of the other glands, pressure massage on the response area for the pituitary as shown in Chart 2A, will start correcting the problem right away. Pressure massage on this response area every once-in-awhile for nine minutes will help keep your entire system functioning properly and insure you good health for years to come.

THE PINEAL

The pineal gland is a small conical organ, lying at about the middle of the brain. If it malfunctions many things can happen. For example, the sex glands develop prematurely, and the other glands' activities and development are also upset. Apply pressure massage to the response area for the pineal gland just above that of the pituitary as shown in Chart 2A to restore balance to this all important gland.

SWELLING

Edema is a condition where the body tissues retain abnormal amounts of fluid due to an upset in the osmotic pressures of the tissues. This gives you a very puffy appearance. It is caused many times by too much salt intake into the body, which upsets the potassium-sodium balance. Also, if the pituitary and pineal glands are malfunctioning, this balance is also upset. Pressure massage on the response areas for the pituitary and pineal glands on the bottom of the big toe as shown in Chart 2A will readjust this balance and keep your osmotic pressure in order.

A CASE OF EDEMA

Mr. N. came to me hoping for permanent help in the recurring swelling that had kept him in and out of a hospital for two years. He was overweight and compounded his problem by eating all of the wrong things. Pizza, donuts, candy, potato chips and pop were staples in his diet. Everything he ate was drowned in salt. His kidneys were overburdened by this continued ingestion of the wrong foods.

The idea that his diet had anything to do with his condition was a surprise to him. He was willing to try anything so he agreed to remove salt and pastries from his diet. A diet of fresh, raw fruits and vegetables immediately relieved the burden of his weakened kidneys.

Pointed Pressure Massage twice weekly on the response areas for the entire glandular system began to restore balance to his system. We found the pituitary, adrenal, and heart response areas particularly tender. He became aquainted with the massage technique and continued the treatment for nearly six months. At his annual check up, I couldn't find a trace of his previous problems. Even his heart had returned to normal.

FATIGUE

Many common diseases have their origin in the malfunctioning of one or more of the endocrine glands. For example, who would think that the common problem of fatigue would be associated with a glandular problem and not merely overwork or lack of rest? Chronic fatigue is often associated with congestion in the thyroid and adrenal glands. Also the pituitary gland can add to the feeling of always being tired, if it is not functioning properly. Pointed Pressure Massage of the response areas to these glands, as well as to the sex glands, will start to pick you up.

A QUICK PICKUP

A quick pick-me-up can be had by massaging the adrenals as shown in Chart 2A for nine minutes. If you feel tired all the time and the littlest tasks seem like a lot of work, chances are the response areas to your glands, particularly the thyroid, pituitary and adrenals need massaging twice a week for nine minutes at a time until the tenderness of the response area is gone.

SLEEP WITHOUT PILLS

Another common problem often associated with fatigue is insomnia. This is a chronic inability to sleep, or if you do go to sleep you wake up often and find it hard to go back to sleep. Many times you will be so tired you can't seem to go to sleep without a sleeping pill. With Pointed Pressure Massage this is no longer necessary. The problem exists in a malfunctioning of the thyroid gland or sex reflexes. Treatment by pressure massage for both these glands, particularly the thyroid will begin to help you get to sleep. Also before you go to bed, massage the response area for general relaxation as shown in Chart 2A, for nine minutes. This will relax you and enable you to fall asleep much faster than usual.

A CASE OF INSOMNIA AND FATIGUE CURED

Mr. D. was spending half the night reading in an attempt to get to sleep. When he did finally get to sleep it lasted for only two to four hours. He had used sleeping pills until he was afraid they were actually causing side effects without really helping him sleep. He was always tired and felt sleepy during the daytime hours, yet when he tried to take a nap he couldn't get to sleep. When a friend suggested Pointed Pressure Massage for his problem he was eager to give it a try.

First we massaged the response area for general relaxation as shown in Chart 2A, and then we began a series of treatments on the adrenal, thyroid and sex glands. The thyroid response area, which is just under the ball of the foot below the big toe, Chart 2A, was very tender. We gave this area a thorough but brief massage the first time and increased it to a full nine minutes by the third treatment. We then expanded the treatment to applying pressure massage to the response areas for the adrenals, shown in Chart 2A and then for the sex glands. You will find the response area for the sex glands just behind the ankle bone as shown in Chart 6.

After massaging these areas for five weeks, he was beginning to unwind enough to fall asleep before midnight, something he had not been able to do for years. His pep returned and he no longer felt tired 24 hours a day. Having learned how and where to massage the proper areas for his sluggish condition he has been able to prevent the problem from returning.

ALLERGIES

Allergies are due to many diverse things such as chemicals, food, animals, pollen, reactions to cold and hot, sun, clothing, and many more. They are also caused by an imbalance in the glandular system. If you are bothered by allergies of any kind and in any way, gently apply pressure massage on the bottom of your feet in the areas of the endocrine glands as shown in Chart 2A, to locate tender response areas. These tender areas are associated with malfunctioning glands. They should be massaged twice a week, nine minutes at a time until the tenderness is gone.

BLOOD SUGAR

High and low blood sugar, due to a malfunctioning of the pancreas, can cause allergic attacks. Also an imbalance of potassium and sodium in the system can cause allergies. Pressure massage on the particular glands that are misfunctioning will alleviate allergies without the addition of pills and drugs to the system. Nature made her own way to cure problems without the use of drugs. Application of pressure massage will convince you that her way is truly the best.

HAY FEVER

Hayfever, a specific type of allergy, causes millions of people discomfort during the pollen season. Even with all pressure massage can do to lessen the suffering, it can not be completely done away with if the pollen causing the allergy is in the air. Pressure massage applied to the endocrine glands, particularly the thyroid and pancreas shown in Charts 2A and 2B can make things bearable again. The important thing to remember here, is that many people with hayfever develop asthma and this can be very serious. With pressure massage, hayfever itself can be lessened and asthma can be prevented. This will be discussed more fully under "Help for the Asthmatic" in Chapter 15.

SLOW THE AGING PROCESS

Chronological age cannot be slowed down, but the degeneration of the physical body can be miraculously slowed by pressure massage on the entire endocrine glands. Rejuvenation measures should be used before signs develop indicating a rapid slowing of the physical processes. Instead of relying on drug replacement therapies such as estrogen and androgen, a comprehensive program of pressure massage on the response areas of the appropriate glands should be instigated. A soreness in the response area indicates that the gland needs rejuvenation. General pressure massage of the response areas for all glands, Chart 2A, as well as the liver, Chart 4, will begin rejuvenation and slow degeneration.

SENILITY

Reduced functioning of the glandular system can lead to senility. This can cause a weakness of the mental and/or physical body. Often it sets in before it really should because of a glandular disorder. Massaging the response areas to the glands can overcome much of the weakness, or head it off before it sets in.

CONVULSIONS

Epilepsy, an episodic disturbance of consciousness during which convulsions may occur, is often caused by a head injury. Many times the problem is simply due to an imbalance in the glandular system. By massaging the response areas for the entire endocrine glands, seizures may be lessened and medication may be eliminated. This depends though upon the type and intensity of epilepsy. Pressure massage will lessen the seizures in every case and if a person is in an attack it will bring them out after a few minutes. If you are an epileptic or know someone that is one, find the tender response areas on the bottom of your feet for the glands and begin treatment on them right away. Also remember these areas if a seizure comes on. Pressure massage will lead you to good health if you only give it a try.

A CASE OF EPILEPSY CONTROLLED

After years of taking drugs to suppress his attacks, Mr. B. was having more attacks with greater severity. By applying pressure massage to the response areas for the endocrine glands twice weekly for six months his attacks had been reduced to one every four to six weeks. He became interested in massaging the response areas for the glands himself so I gave him a chart which located the pineal, pituitary, thyroid, parathyroid, pancreas, adrenals and the sex organs. Massaging these areas regularly over a period of several years enabled him to go as long as three months without an attack. The frequency and the severity of his attacks were also reduced. He feels that if he had been able to use this massage years earlier he could have avoided the use of drugs and possibly cleared up the problem entirely.

METABOLISM

Another problem which occurs within the digestive and circulatory systems but is dependent on glandular functioning is that of metabolism. It is the sum of all physical and chemical processes by which a living organized substance is produced and maintained, and also is the transformation by which energy is made available for the use of the organism. In other words it is the sum of all processes which keep us functioning as living organisms. Proper metabolism is vital to a healthy existence. Keeping the glands healthy and functioning properly will insure good metabolism. Pointed Pressure Massage on the response areas to the thyroid, pancreas and pituitary glands as shown in Chart 2B will help metabolism to continue to maintain a healthy state.

YOUR GLANDULAR TEAM

As you can see by now the endocrine glands work together as a team to maintain the equilibrium necessary for healthy living. Many times if one gland is malfunctioning all the other glands will be involved and also often be malfunctioning as well. Pointed Pressure Massage to the entire system can and will combat upsets in the whole body and you will feel like you were created to feel — Good and Healthy.

DIABETES

Mrs. Y. had gorged herself for many years and had been as much as 100 lbs. overweight. All of the complaints associated with overweight people were hers and she finally decided to do something about it. She was constantly hungry, had to urinate frequently, was always thirsty, mentally depressed and had a dry, red tongue.

TREATMENT:

Pressure therapy to the response area for the pancreas as shown on Charts 2A and 2B and a correction of the diet. In the case of diabetes, rarely does one improve without the benefit of both pressure therapy and a revision of the diet. The diet must be converted entirely to raw fruits and vegetables for a period of approximately six months — the first three months should be almost entirely of fresh raw vegetables and or juices with the addition of raw fruits the second three months. During this time those taking insulin should gradually reduce the amount as tests indicate it should be reduced. Never should the use of insulin be stopped abruptly — only on a gradual basis when the tests indicate less need for it and on the advice of a doctor.

LENGTH OF TREATMENT:

Since it takes so long to drop weight safely I give pressure therapy only once a week to allow the recuperative ability of the body to correct the abnormal condition of the pancreas and restore balance to the kidneys and digestive system. Depending on the severity of the case — the amount of overweight — treatment runs for six months to a year. Mrs. Y. continued for 14 months at which time she no longer needed insulin. Eight years later she is on a maintanence diet and feels fine.

chapter 9

Helping Your
Disease Fighters With
Pressure Therapy

The lymphatic system is a closed system like the blood vascular system but the walls of the lymphatic vessels are thinner and more permeable than those of the blood capillaries. It consists of lymph capillaries, lymphatic vessels, lymphatic ducts and lymph nodes.

Lymph is a fluid quite similar to blood plasma except that it has a large number of white blood cells, mostly lymphocytes, and only a few red blood cells. Lymph also clots very slowly.

LYMPH VESSELS

Lymph vessels have three major functions. They return to the blood vessels vital substances, chiefly proteins, which have leaked out into the capillary beds. Also they provide drainage channels into lymph nodes for toxic or malignant materials. The lymphatic vessels in the intestines are important in the absorption of digested fats.

LYMPH NODES

The lymph nodes have many functions also. They filter and, to a large degree, quarantine the noxious products of inflammation or malignant lesions. Also, they produce lymphocytes and release them into the blood. They function in producing immunity to diseases and transplanted tissues.

As you can see the lymphatic system is very important in preventing an invasion of the blood by bacteria or other germs, which are usually filtered out in the lymph nodes and ingested by the white cells. Lymphatic vessels occur in nearly all parts and organs of the body except in the brain and spinal cord. Since it is so widespread in the body, the lymphatic system is an ideal route for the spread of infection which has become so serious it can no longer be controlled by the white cells and the lymph nodes. An infection such as this can easily get into the blood stream and spread all over the body in a few hours.

Viruses can also be dangerous because they can pass through the lymph nodes without any trouble. The lymphatic system is equally important in the spread of cancer cells from one organ or part of the body to another.

There are three organs closely related to the lymphatic system. They are the spleen, the tonsils-adenoids and the thymus.

THE SPLEEN

The spleen is a soft, dark brownish-red organ lying along the greater curvature of the stomach. It is the largest mass of lymphatic tissue in the body. In proportion to its size it has one of the richest blood supplies of any organ in the body.

This organ is very important in the body's defense against disease, since it manufactures lymphocytes and antibodies. It also destroys old worn-out and abnormal red blood cells and the platelet cells of the blood. The spleen acts as a reservoir for blood which can very rapidly be poured out into the circulatory system if needed in an emergency. Another function of the spleen as a defense mechanism, is that of filtering microorganisms from the blood.

Any diseases which affect the spleen can profoundly affect several important body functions also. It is therefore very important for your spleen to stay healthy. This can be assured with Pointed Pressure Massage. Since the spleen lies along the stomach, massaging the response areas to the stomach will keep not only the stomach and pancreas healthy but also the spleen. See Chart 2B.

TONSILS—ADENOIDS

The tonsils are organs which form a ring of lymphatic tissue around the entrances of the alimentary and respiratory tract and thus protect them from the invasion of bacteria. One of these pair of organs is called the adenoids. They are often enlarged in infants and adults.

The tonsils form a protective barrier for the mouth, throat, larynx, trachea and lungs. They are also important in the development of immune bodies and should not be removed unless completely necessary.

Chronic infection of the tonsils (Tonsillitis) can be very painful. It is an enlargement and tenderness of these organs. This is caused by a general toxification of the entire body, a bad diet, too much sugar and starch intake, and a deficiency of vitamins. Correction of the diet, addition of vitamins A, C, and D and a faithful application of pressure massage can and will eliminate any trouble with the tonsils and adenoids. It must be remembered that troubles within the tonsils and adenoids do not go away over night and perseverance in treatment is required.

HELP FOR SORE TONSILS

There are response areas for the tonsils on the feet (see Chart 2B). Pressure massage on these areas for nine minutes a day every other day (more often if your problem is acute) will help you restore health to your tonsils and in a little time the recurrent soreness will disappear. Also pressure massage on the response areas for the throat on the hands as shown in Chart 2B will relieve that sore, scratchy throat that often accompanies soreness in the tonsils.

TONSILITIS CURED

Mrs. B. had reoccurring throat infections from grade school through high school. When she went to college this came to the attention of the nurse who immediately suggested the removal of the tonsils and adenoids. An arrangement was made for the operation to be done at the expense of the college health services. Shortly before the day of the operation she became ill and the operation was postponed. The new date was never set because of the end of the school year.

The following year she was married and the infections popped up frequently during the next few years. When a particularly severe infection caused her to be out of work for a week she came to me for help hoping to avoid that word "surgery."

I found the response area for the throat on the hand between the thumb and the first finger Chart 5 to be very tender. We applied Pointed Pressure Massage to these areas for three consecutive days, at which time she could swallow with only little difficulty. On the fifth day the swelling and soreness were gone but the response areas remained tender. I instructed her to massage these areas twice weekly until they were no longer tender and to come back for a check-up in six weeks.

At the next check-up all the tenderness was gone and her tonsils and adenoids appeared normal. They have remained normal for the ensuing 20 years. She has had no sore throats or swelling of the tonsils and her general health has been excellent.

Your tonsils and adenoids are there for a purpose. Do not have them removed until you have first tried Pointed Pressure Massage. I have never had a case of bad tonsils that pressure massage would not correct.

A word of caution — do not confuse enlarged tonsils with strep throat. Strep throat can be deadly and requires medical attention immediately.

THE THYMUS

The thymus is a flat, pinkish-gray, two-lobed organ lying high in the chest slightly above the heart. It is relatively large in infants but regresses in size after puberty and atropies. This ductless gland is one of the central controls of the body's immunity system. How it works is not completely understood. It is thought that the thymus serves to supply fresh lymphocytes to lymphatic tissue for the purpose of reacting against new antigens, in other words it forms antibodies. What is known is that a healthy thymus is vital in proper adjustment of adolescents.

Problems occurring in the lymph glands are usually infections, inflammation and toxins in the system due to diseased organs or an internal infection. The use of too much table salt often causes or compounds the problems. Its use must be eliminated. Pressure massage on the response areas of the lymph glands as shown in Chart 6 for nine minutes every 3rd day will insure proper functioning of this system. Your fight against disease is dependent on the health of this entire system and its organs. Take care of it and it will take care of you.

SOME IMPORTANT NOTES
ABOUT OUR DISEASE FIGHTERS

The rush of needless surgery in the past 20 years has left us with a generation prone to disease and dysfunction. Could anyone believe that the body came equipped with needless organs or superfluous appendages? The tonsils, adenoids, and the appendix were there for the purpose of fighting disease but millions have been removed because their functions were misunderstood.

The tonsils act as a filter to prevent the body from invasion of bacteria and aid in the formation of white cells. Their removal lowers the body's ability to prevent infection of the respiratory system and also upsets the ability to regulate the production of white blood cells. Many anemia problems arise from the loss of this regulator. Future research may link leukemia to the needless removal of tonsils.

If you still have your adenoids and tonsils, keep them. Any temporary infection you may have can be removed by gargling every 15 minutes with a very weak solution of vinegar and water for 24 hours. The tonsils may be returned to normal size then by applying Pointed Pressure Massage to the response area for the tonsils as shown in Chart 2A for nine minutes twice weekly until all swelling is gone.

The vermiform appendix should not be removed unless it has ruptured or rupturing is imminent. For many years it was needlessly removed because it was considered by many to be useless. It is now known to be a germ fighter for the intestinal tract and a blow off valve for excessive pressure in the intestines. The reason for removal lies in the failure to understand its function and, more specifically, in not knowing how to relieve it without surgery. I have relieved many cases by simply applying pressure massage to the response areas for the appendix as shown in Chart 2A. A case history for this is described in the section concerned with digestion. The Bunching technique described in Chapter 5 is very useful in the case of appendicitis.

SORE THROATS

Jayne L. had sore throats for years after she had her tonsils removed. She didn't have sinus problems but very frequently the soreness went down to the bronchial area and several times into the lungs.

TREATMENT:

Pressure Therapy between the thumb and first finger as shown on Chart 5 for nine minutes every other day for one week checked the immediate sore throat and prevented the inflammation from going down into the lung area.

LENGTH OF TREATMENT:

During this week we began teaching her to apply this pressure for herself and advised her to spend a little time on one hand or the other for a period of two months. We also increased her vitamin C intake to 600 mg per day — the level at which she began losing some in the urine tests indicating that was the most she could utilize. Three months later she was ready to start into the coming winter hopeful the "sore throat" period would pass her by. For the most part it did although she did have one seige this winter — mild compared to previous winters. In the successive three winters she was free from the ravages of the sore throats she had been accustomed to having.

chapter 10

How To Cure
That Aching Back

The musculo-skeletal system consists of the muscles and the bones of the body. Within the body, muscles and bones work together for protection, support and movement. Many common problems with the back and neck are due to problems within the muscles and bones together or sometimes separately. Usually they cannot be separated and both must be worked on for complete relief.

MUSCLES

The muscles provide the power for the movement of parts of the body. They are attached to the bones by tendons. Muscles can only contract or shorten, which causes pulling on the places where it is attached to the bones. For this reason most of the muscles are arranged in antagonistic pairs on the opposite sides of a movable joint. When one muscle of the pair contracts, it moves a part of the body in one direction and its antagonistic (opposite) muscle when it contracts moves the part in the opposite direction.

Within our bodies a muscle very rarely acts alone. It nearly always acts in association with other muscles as a group. Because of this when we have a sore muscle we usually have several closely associated ones that are also sore. Muscles act in an orderly fashion. To perform even the slightest movement every muscle involved must cooperate. The result of cooperation is coordination, which is vital to life. If a muscle becomes paralyzed, coordination is disrupted. This effects other muscles as well as the one that is paralyzed. Atrophy can set in if the condition is not corrected.

There are around 327 paired and two unpaired skeletal muscles in the body. They make up nearly half of the total body tissue of a normal adult. The muscular tissue is called a skeletal muscle because it is attached to some part of the skeleton. It is also called voluntary muscle because it is under the control of our will except in diseased cases.

DISORDERS OF THE MUSCLES

Problems within the muscles usually originate in the nerve supply, the blood supply or within the connective tissue of the muscle. Symptoms of disorders are paralysis, weakness, pain, atrophy, spasms, and cramps.

CHARLEY HORSE — CRAMPS

Did you ever get a cramp in your foot that you couldn't get out? Cramps can be very painful and annoying. With

Pointed Pressure Massage they need not ever bother you again. Since cramps can occur in the muscles of the arms, legs, feet, hands and heart, you must apply pressure massage on their particular response areas. You then can relieve their pain and eliminate them completely. The response areas are as follows: For the arm you apply pressure massage on the leg as shown in Chart 3. For the leg you massage the arm which is also shown in Chart 5. For the foot you work on the hands as shown in Chart 5, and for the heart you massage the response area for the heart on the left foot as shown in Chart 2B.

A CASE OF CRAMPS RELIEVED

Mr. L. began having severe cramps in the legs following an infection of the throat which had been diagnosed as strep throat. The use of sulfa drugs during this illness had destroyed the beneficial bacteria of the intestines commonly known as the intestinal flora. Without this normal digestive factor he was unable to assimilate some of the nutrients from his food such as the B vitamins. Over a period of weeks this led to a weakened nervous system which became apparent in the form of muscle spasms and severe cramps. When they became very severe and uncontrollable he came looking for relief. By applying Pointed Pressure Massage on the response area for the muscles on the middle finger for nine minutes and the response area for the leg on the arm for nine minutes we relieved the charley horse that had been unbearable for so many hours.

This treatment was continued every other day for three weeks during which time he became familiar with the areas to massage until he recovered completely. With the addition of the B vitamins and yogurt to his diet the beneficial bacteria of the digestive tract were brought back to a normal balance. A check-up six months later showed complete recovery.

MUSCULAR PAIN

Muscular pain can be caused by several things such as overwork or exercise, sickness, injury or a release of too much poison at one time so that the kidneys and sweat glands cannot remove it right away. Problems with back muscles in general can be treated by applying pressure massage to the second finger on the hands as shown in Chart 3.

BACK TROUBLE

It seems in our modern society that back trouble is a very common problem. It is shared by men and women alike. Some causes could be the lack of exercise, a poor posture, a deficiency of minerals, a sagging bed, or an injury. Yes, a sagging bed is a very common cause of back aches. Usually a piece of plywood between the mattresses will solve the problem. Besides this correction, your diet and posture may need to be changed and an addition of the trace minerals may be required.

Back problems are classified three ways according to their location.

LOWER BACK

The first type is that of the lower back or lumbago. This can be very painful and usually makes it so you cannot bend over. There are about three major response areas for lumbago. First apply pressure massage to the palm of the hands including the palmar surface of the thumb and fingers as shown in Chart 3. I have found the easiest way to apply this pressure evenly and adequately is to take an ordinary metal comb and press the teeth firmly on the palm area for 10 to 20 minutes daily moving it over the surface while continuing to press firmly. The second response area is that of the web between the thumb and the first finger and the web between the first and second finger on both hands. Chart 5. Massage these areas with your hands for nine minutes daily. The third response area is that of the base of the spine on the feet as shown in Chart 2A. This area should also be massaged for nine minutes at a time.

I suggest the comb treatment every day for 10 to 20 minutes and alternating the other two treatments for best results.

A CASE OF LUMBAGO HELPED

Mr. J. began having pains in the lower back area when he was forced to take a shipping dock position because of a company setback. For over 10 years he had done only desk work and no manual labor. He could remember no particular reason for the back ache. There hadn't been any falls or strains in lifting and he could find little to explain the increasing pain. Over the years he had added over 40 pounds to his weight and his posture was far from being ideal. Spinal X-rays showed no dislocated or broken vertebrae. A check on the response areas for the lower back revealed a muscle imbalance on the right side which was causing the discomfort. By massaging the response area for the lower back located on the palm and between the thumb and first finger, we relieved the pain so that he could stand erect without discomfort. Further treatment on the response area located on the foot for the spine completed the return to normalcy. A planned program for weight reduction was reducing the load on his spinal column and improving his chances of keeping a healthy back.

SHOULDERS

The second type of back trouble involves the muscles of the shoulders and the upper back. Shoulder trouble can cause a lot of pain and is many times caused by tension and strain.

With pressure massage you can alleviate this pain and relax those shoulder muscles. Just apply pressure massage to the response area for the shoulders on your foot for nine minutes a day. This response area is on the outer edge of the bottom of the foot as shown in Chart 2A. Sit down in a comfortable position and apply pressure to this response area and get rid of those aching shoulders yourself — without aspirin or other drugs.

BACK OF THE NECK

The third major type of back trouble involves that of the muscles of the back of the neck and the muscles of the back in the neck area. Soreness and stiffness in the neck is also due to nervous strain and tension.

If you have ever suffered from a stiff (wry) neck you know the pain and inconvenience of it. Thank goodness relief is only 10 minutes away. The response areas are located on the hands and feet as shown in Chart 2A.

CASE OF A WRY NECK

Reverend P. was most skeptical of any connection between the bottom of his feet and his stiff (wry) neck, but when all else had failed and the pain grew to where he could hardly stand it, he requested a pressure massage treatment.

I began the treatment by having him sit down in a comfortable position as I started to massage the bottom of his feet. The response area for the back of the neck on the big toe as shown in Chart 2A was very tender. I applied pressure massage for nine minutes after which he decided to try and turn his neck. To his complete amazement Rev. P. noted that he could now move his head without any discomfort at all. This was the first time he had been able to do so for weeks and he wanted to immediately go and show his wife.

THE BONES

There are over 200 bones in the body which constitute about 20% of the body tissue of an adult. The skelton is divided into an axial and an appendicular part. The axial part consists of the skull, the face and cranium; the hyoid located in the throat; the vertebral column; the 12 pairs of ribs and the sternum or breast bone. The appendicular part consists of the pectoral (shoulder) girdle with the scapula (shoulder blade) and the clavicle (collar bone); the pelvic girdle (hip bones) with the sacrum; and the bones of the arms and legs.

The bones of the body have many important functions. They serve as support for the various organs of the body and enable us to stand. Also they serve as levers and points of attachment for the muscles. Without them movement would be impossible.

In addition to all these functions is that of protection which is really the most important for survival. Our brain and spinal cord are surrounded and protected by the bones of the skull and vertebrae. Our heart, lungs, liver, stomach, and spleen are protected by the ribs and breast bone. Within the pelvis our bladder, rectum, and internal reproductive organs are also protected. You can see how important bones really are. Without them the proper functioning of our bodies would be impossible.

OSTEOPOROSIS

Osteoporosis, a degeneration of the bone is a very serious disease of the skeletal system. It is caused by a depletion of proper glandular activity, inadequate supplies of vitamins and calcium intake. You must add vitamins A and D, the trace minerals (dolomite) and calcium (bone meal) to your diet if you want to head off this problem. Then Pointed Pressure Massage can help you. Apply pressure massage to the response areas for the entire endocrine glands as shown in Charts 2A and 2B. Treatments for nine minutes a day every 3rd day until the tenderness of the response areas is gone will ensure you of healthy bones again.

LENGTHENING A SHORT LEG

At the age of nine years Miss D. jumped off the front porch, a drop of some eleven inches, and landed on the heel of her right foot. Three months later her mother brought her to me because she was apparently developing a condition of one leg becoming shorter than the other. She limped and said it hurt to walk.

An examination revealed that her pelvis had been tipped and thus dislocated by the jump and she was getting worse daily. Standard medical treatment for this is to elevate the heel of the short leg. That procedure is not followed with the system of pressure massage. After massaging the response area to lengthen a short leg as shown in Chart 5 for two months, her leg was returned to a completely normal condition. A way of determining this was to have her stand on two bathroom scales, one foot on each, and note that the weight was distributed evenly (within five pounds) on the scales. We think this is much better than a lifetime of pain and discomfort with a raised heel on one shoe.

Many times a dislocation of joints can cause a short leg or arm etc. Pressure massage can relocate the dislocated joint and thus lengthen the arm or leg so that it will be normal again.

SUBLUXATED VERTEBRAE
CORRECTED BEFORE THE SPINE FUSED

Mr. Y. was accustomed to manual labor and prided himself in his physical stamina. To his astonishment he woke up one morning with a pain in his back that was so severe he could hardly get out of bed. He had lifted more than usual the day before and thought he had only pulled some muscle too hard. When the pain continued for a week keeping him from work he came for help.

We found the response area for the lower back on his instep near his heel, Chart 2A, to be very tender. Pointed Pressure Massage for nine minutes twice a day for three days relaxed the strain on his back and allowed the vertebrae to slip back in place the next night as he slept.

This prevented what could have been years of back trouble which many times causes spinal deterioration and even eventual fusing of the spine at the point of subluxation.

chapter 11

How To Cope
With Nervous Problems

The nervous system consists of specialized cells called neurons, their processes and reception and transmission of nerve stimuli. The neurons are divided up into two parts: the cell bodies, located within or close to the brain and spinal cord and the cell processes which form the nerves throughout the body.

Nerve fibers that bring impulses to the brain or spinal cord are called sensory or afferent fibers. Those fibers that take impulses away from the brain and spinal cord are the motor or efferent fibers. Most nerves contain both types of fibers, but one type usually is predominant.

The nerve impulses coming into the brain or spinal cord arise from stimuli producing sensations of pain, temperature, touch, pressure, taste, sight, sound, smell or the position of the body and its parts. The structures which respond initially to the stimuli producing any of these sensations are the receptors. The receptors for smell, taste, sight, sound, and touch are the special sense organs and will be discussed further in Chapter 16.

The nervous system is a functioning unit for integrating the functions of the other systems of the body and acquainting us with our environment. It, in association with the endocrine system, makes life possible in a changing environment. These systems must be functioning properly if you are to be healthy.

DIVISIONS OF THE NERVOUS SYSTEM

The nervous system is divided into a central and a peripheral nervous system.

THE CENTRAL NERVOUS SYSTEM

The central nervous system consists of the brain and the spinal cord. Within the tissues surrounding the brain and spinal cord and in the cavities of the brain is a fluid called cerebrospinal fluid. In suspected injuries or damages to the CNS some of this fluid may be removed for examination. This fluid cushions the brain and spinal cord and absorbs shock.

THE SPINAL CORD

The vertebrae or spinal column as it is called surrounds and protects the spinal cord which is located in the back of the body running from the bottom of the brain down to the lumbar vertebrae. The spinal cord is approximately 18 inches long which is shorter than the spinal column. It consists of nerve cells and fibers transmitting nerve impulses up and down the cord between the brain and spinal cord.

Injuries or diseases within the spinal cord are very serious. Many problems can be helped with pressure massage if the cord itself is in tack.

SUBLUXATED VERTEBRAE

A subluxated vertebrae is one that is partially dislocated. This can be extremely painful and very serious if it causes a nerve to be pinched. Pointed Pressure Massage will clear this problem up in two to three treatments. You just apply pressure massage to the response areas for the spine as shown in Charts 2A and 2B for nine minutes each treatment. Another method of applying pressure massage for problems in the back is that of massaging the vertebrae directly. This is where you intermittently apply pressure to the area of the subluxated vertebrae with the sides of your hands in an up and down motion very rapidly. This can be thought of as a series of gentle karate chops.

DETERIORATION OR INFLAMMATION
OF THE MYELIN SHEATH

In the case of a deterioration or inflammation of the myelin sheath of a nerve fiber, pressure massage will offer relief. The symptoms of myelitis, which is the common name for this disorder, are a moderate fever, loss of appetite, a coated tongue, constipation and pain in the back which moves to the limbs. There is often numbness, tingling, burning and paralysis may develop if it is not taken care of immediately. Treatment includes applying pressure massage to the response areas for the entire spine as shown also in Charts 2A and 2B. Multiple Sclerosis is a specific type of this deterioration and the treatment is the same as for myelitis.

PARALYSIS

Myelitis is only one cause of paralysis which is a complete loss of the motor functions or movement. If this is due to an impinged nerve, pressure massage can restore the proper functioning.

INFANTILE PARALYSIS

Mrs. J. was stricken with paralysis and was left with partial paralysis on the right side. She could walk but with a decided limp. The right leg was not developing as it should so it was becoming more noticeable each year that she limped. After four years she was brought to my office for an examination. Since this was not a case of complete loss of function there was some nerve supply which had not been cut off. The response area for paralysis on the lobe of the right ear (Chart 4) was very tender and the response area on the back wall of the pharynx was also tender. We applied pressure massage to the ear lobe and using a probe applied pressure massage also to the back wall of the pharynx. Improvement was slow at first but results were positive and after six months complete use was restored. The leg will always be a bit smaller than the other because the paralysis had been allowed to remain for over four years before we began treatment. Had we begun four years earlier not a trace of the problem would have remained. Fortunately the residual effects are so slight that only her closest confidants will know and then only because she may tell them.

THE BRAIN

The other major part of the central nervous system is the brain. It is divided up into three main parts.

THE CEREBRUM

The first main portion is the cerebrum which consists of a right and left part called cerebral hemispheres. Each hemisphere is further divided into four lobes: the frontal, parietal, occipital and temporal. The frontal lobe controls voluntary movements of small groups of muscles and parts of the opposite side of the body. The right hemisphere controls the left side of the body and vice versa. Also associated with the frontal lobe is the control of emotional feelings, accurate judgement, abstract ideas and coordinated movements of the eyes and head. Mental capacity is a function of the cerebral cortex as a whole rather than any particular area.

The parietal lobe lies on the top and side of the cerebrum behind the frontal lobe. It is primarily concerned with touch, pain, temperature, pressure, and position sense from the skin, muscles, and joints of the opposite side of the body. Also, it is concerned with movement of parts of the limbs (hands and fingers) and turning the head and eyes to the opposite side.

The temporal lobe, located below the parietal and frontal lobes, houses the primary center for hearing and language formation. If there is an injury to this area speech defects, ringing or buzzing ears, impairment of memory, epileptic-like seizures, hallucinations, and disturbances in the sense of smell or taste may result.

At the back of the cerebrum is the occipital lobe, often called the visual area of the brain. Injury in this area can cause blindness even though the eyes are perfectly normal.

THE CEREBELLUM

The second main portion of the brain is the cerebellum which is located below the cerebrum. Its chief functions are posture control and coordination of voluntary muscular movements. The cerebellum controls muscular movements of the same side of the body whereas the cerebrum controls that of the opposite sides.

THE BRAIN STEM

The third major portion of the brain is the brain stem. Most of the cranial nerves arise or end in the brain stem. It is the relay station for nerve fibers and tracts passing between the various parts of the brain and the spinal cord. The respiratory center for the control of breathing is also in the brain stem as well as the control of the origin and propagation of the peristaltic waves of the digestive tract.

Problems within the brain include inflammation, tumors, nerve starvation, paralysis, cerebral palsy, depression, emotional problems, memory losses, poor mental health, and stammering. You must remember that the endocrine and nervous systems work together to maintain a balance within our system. If something is wrong with one of these areas it will affect the other as well as many other parts of the body.

CEREBRAL PALSY

Cerebral palsy is a type of paralysis due to impairment of the nerves by a blood clot or tumor in the cerebrum. If it is caused by a blood clot you can immediately begin to lower the blood pressure by applying pressure massage to the response area for circulation as shown in Chart 4. Also apply pressure on the soft palate in the back of the mouth with a rounded spoon.

MEMORY

In problems with memory, pressure massage on the response areas for memory on the sides of the forehead as shown in Chart 4 can stimulate your cerebrum and thus give your memory new vitality.

MENTAL HEALTH

Our emotions and mental health are very important to us if we are to be healthy individuals. Depression is a common emotional manifestation and is many times due to a mal-functioning in our nervous or endocrine systems. Often these problems are caused by bad diet, little rest, and deficiencies in vitamins. If this is corrected, pressure massage will do the rest for you. Massage response areas for general relaxation as shown in Chart 2A; mental health and nerves Chart 4; the back of the neck and shoulders Chart 2A; the endocrine glands Chart 2A and the brain Chart 3. Alternate daily over all these response areas working nine minutes on one, one day and nine minutes on a different one the next day. Remember a healthy mental state can insure a healthy body.

STAMMERING

Stammering is caused by a disruptive nerve balance to the brain and is many times accompanied by a subluxated vertebrae in the cervical region. It can in practically every case be eliminated with pressure massage. Begin treatment by massaging the response area for stammering on the lower part of the back of the neck as shown in Chart 5. To get the subluxated vertebrae back in place, apply pressure with the sides of your hands in a rapid up and down motion, to the cervical area of the vertebrae.

STAMMERING NEED NOT BOTHER YOU

Mr. V. was a very nervous lad. At twelve years of age he was becoming tired of being the object of so much ridicule and cutting jokes about his speech problem. Sometimes, when there was very little emotional stress, he could talk quite freely without stuttering. Any excitement would suddenly cause him to have difficulty speaking.

An examination revealed two things which caused him to have a serious shortage of the B vitamins. He ate a typical candy and starch diet so many young people live on today. In addition to this he had a hypermobile intestine which caused the further loss of B vitamins when the food passed through the system too fast.

We suggested a correction in the eating habits and worked on the response areas for the stomach and intestines shown in Chart 2A, to restore the normal functions to this area. Simultaneously we worked on the response area for stammering as shown in Chart 5 in the neck area. In three months time his digestive tract was functioning properly and he was having less trouble with his speech. By the time school was out he was no longer bothered by speech problems.

THE PERIPHERAL NERVOUS SYSTEM

The peripheral nervous system consists of the cranial and spinal nerves as well as the autonomic nervous system. Its function is primarily the conduction of nerve impulses to and from the central nervous system.

CRANIAL NERVES

There are 12 pairs of cranial nerves which all arise from the brain within the skull except for the olfactory nerve. They function for the sense of smell, taste, sight, hearing, balance, movement of the eyes, and the movement of the muscles to the jaw, pharynx, larynx, abdominal organs and the tongue.

THE AUTONOMIC NERVOUS SYSTEM

The autonomic nervous system is further divided into two subdivisions. The parasympathetic fibers and the sympathetic fibers. Stimulation of the parasympathetic fibers produces actions of slowing the heart beat and secretions of the glands, constriction (closing) of the pupil and bronchial tubes, increased mobility of the intestines, contraction of the bladder, dilation of the blood vessels of the salivary glands, brain and external sex organs. The sympathetic system does just the opposite. It alone supplies the blood vessels of the skin, muscles, abdominal and pelvic organs, sweat glands, liver and adrenal glands.

NEURITIS

Neuritis is nerve starvation which results in the inflammation of the nerves. This can be caused by pinched nerves, bad diets, and vitamin deficiency. Add vitamins B-complex and C and the trace minerals to your diet and apply pressure massage to the hands with rubber bands. This can be done by wrapping a rubber band around the last joint of each finger and leaving them on for nine minutes at a time. Never leave them on over eleven minutes.

STAMMERING

Bob S. had stammered ever since he was a young child. Treatment followed treatment for years until finally the family decided it was useless. When he came to me for a back injury from college football practice, I asked him if he would like the stammering cleared up while I was working on his back. He said he had tried everything but as long as he was here, to go ahead.

TREATMENT:

The treatment for his back lasted four weeks during which time I applied pressure therapy to the response area for stammering shown on Chart 5.

By the end of the fourth week his back had returned to normal and he was doing less stammering.

We made a mark on his back at the response area for stammering so he could have members of his family apply the pressure during the summer. When he returned in the fall he was free of his stammering and is still free fifteen years later.

chapter 12

Pressure Therapy
Can Restore Balance
of Sex Organs

The reproductive system consists of those organs used in reproduction of life and those concerned with the sex characteristics of the male and female. It is divided into the male reproductive system and the female reproductive system.

THE MALE REPRODUCTORY ORGANS

The internal organs of the male reproductive system are the testi, the epididymis, vas deferens, the prostate gland, the seminal vesicles and the urethra.

The testis (testicle) is a slightly flattened gland about the size and shape of a walnut. It is housed in a sac of skin called the scrotum. Within each testis there are over 800 coiled seminiferous tubules which form the sperm or male sex cells.

Besides being important in the reproductive system, the testis is an important endocrine gland that secretes the male sex hormone — testosterone. This hormone is responsible for the development of secondary sex characteristics such as a beard, pubic and armpit hair and a deeper voice which appear in a boy at the time of puberty. It is also at this time that the formation of the functional sperm appears and therefore the capacity for procreation.

Once the sperm are formed they leave the testis through a duct, the epididymis, a C-shaped structure which lies along the side of each testis. These ducts then empty into a single duct the ductus (vas) deferens which takes the sperm to the urethra, which is a tube-like organ within the penis which transmits both semen with the sperm and urine. Sperm are stored in the epididymis and vas deferens.

Behind the prostate gland and on the base of the urinary bladder are a right and left seminal vesicle. These are hollow sac-like organs whose duct joins the vas deferens to form the ejaculatory duct. The seminal vesicles produce most of the seminal fluid but do not store the sperm.

The prostate gland, a chestnut-like organ, surrounds the first inch of the urethra and secretes an alkaline fluid which aids in the mobility of the sperm cells.

Two common problems that occur within the male reproductive system are hernias and problems with the prostate gland.

HERNIA

A hernia is usually a small loop of intestine or fat which passes through the abdominal wall. It can be very painful and is usually caused by a strain. In many cases a hernia is caused within the newborn by childbirth.

PROSTATE GLAND

In older men a progressive enlargement of the prostate gland commonly obstructs the urethra and thus interferes with the passage of urine. With Pointed Pressure Massage you can reduce the size of the prostate and thus allow the urine to pass freely. Apply pressure massage to the response area for the prostate gland on the side of the foot as shown in Chart 6.

The prostate gland is also a common site for cancer in elderly men. This can be eliminated before it starts by keeping a healthy gland with pressure massage.

PROSTATE — DISEASE OF YOUNG AND OLD
A CASE OF PROSTATE RESTORATION

Mr. L. at 29 years of age was so young he was convinced his problem was his kidneys. He had been told only aging men have prostate troubles. His symptoms could have indicated kidney trouble, painful and frequent urination but it also could have indicated other troubles such as veneral disease. I assured him that we would determine where the problem was and proceeded to examine his feet for tender response areas. The kidneys showed no problem existed there but the prostate gland response areas were so tender you could hardly touch them. We applied Pointed Pressure Massage for only a short time since it was so tender. The results were almost unbelievable. He had a complete nights rest for the first time in six weeks. Treatments every third day for three weeks completely removed his problems. The congestion was gone and with it the problems he thought stemmed from kidney trouble.

You don't have to be bothered with this very annoying and painful condition regardless of your age. Study the location of the response areas carefully and begin your own pressure massage before it gets to the point where you have to look for outside help.

Look at the response area for the prostate. You will notice that it is on the outside of the foot toward the rear and runs parallel with the large tendon at the back of the heel. Firmly press along this area until you locate the exact point where the most tenderness exists. When you have located this spot continue to massage with your thumb or a similar pointed object for at least nine minutes. Repeat the massage every day until all of the tenderness is gone. Usually this will require several weeks and when it is completely normal you will have averted serious and needless surgery.

THE FEMALE REPRODUCTIVE ORGANS

The internal organs of the female reproductive system are the vagina, uterus, uterine tubes and the ovaries.

The ovaries are two oval-shaped structures located in the upper part of the pelvic cavity one on each side of the uterus. They consist of minute follicles (Graafian follicles) which are at various stages of development. The ova or eggs develop within these follicles which rupture at ovulation. The ovaries have two major functions: The development and expulsion of the ova and the production of the female sex hormones. Because of the latter it is an important endocrine gland. One of the hormones produced is estrogen, the female sex hormone which is produced in the Graafian follicles and is responsible for the various changes occurring during the menstrual cycle. It is also responsible for the secondary sex characteristics, enlargement of the breast, pubic and armpit hair and the widening of the hips which occur at puberty.

After the egg leaves the ovary it enters one of the uterine (Fallopian) tubes which takes it to the uterus (womb) by way of muscular contraction and the movement of the cilia within the tubes. The uterus is a hollow pear-shaped organ with thick muscular walls.

Fertilization usually takes place in the Fallopian tubes as the egg is descending to the uterus after ovulation. The sperm work their way up the vagina into the uterus and up to the tubes.

There are many problems associated with the female reproductive organs.

FEMALE DISORDERS

The causes of female disorders include a bad diet, vitamin and mineral deficiencies, an injury and heredity. First you must correct your diet. Remove all white sugar and white flour products and add Vitamins A, B-complex, C, D, and E as well as liver, iron and the trace mineral supplements. After this is done, apply Pointed Pressure Massage and in a few months you will notice a real improvement.

MENSTRUAL CRAMPS

Many women suffer monthly with menstrual cramps. Cramps can be a mild discomfort or a severe crippler. Some women have them so bad that they must remain in bed several hours at a time. This is unnecessary. Do you suffer from cramps? If so there is a treatment which does not involve drugs and pills of any kind. Just apply pressure massage to the response areas for the stomach on the foot as shown in Chart 3, and for the uterus on the foot as shown in Chart 6.

MENSTRUATION SUPPRESSED

If menstruation is suppressed, pressure massage on the base of the tongue and the wall of the pharynx with a cotton-tipped probe or teaspoon will alleviate the problem.

MENOPAUSE

Menopause can be a very hard time for women. There is a drastic change in the hormonal balance and this effects different women in different ways. If you are reaching the age of menopause around 45 to 50 years of age or if you are in menopause, Pointed Pressure Massage can be a big help for you.

Apply pressure to the response areas for the entire endocrine glands on the top of the feet as shown in Charts 2A and 2B. A glandular imbalance always accompanies menstruation and pressure massage will restore this balance. Suggested treatments are for nine minutes every three days.

MISCARRIAGE

A miscarriage can be a very traumatic experience which affects the emotional and physical stability of the body. In case of threatened abortion or false labor, you should rub a wire brush over the back of your hands for several minutes, and repeat this every hour.

Also, put rubber bands on the first joint of each toe (nearest the nail). The bands must be wrapped tightly and left on for nine minutes at a time for the best results. NEVER leave them on for more than eleven minutes because you will cut off the blood circulation.

PREGNANCY

Problems usually associated with pregnancy are morning sickness, vomiting and dizziness. If you have morning sickness, clasp your hands together tightly for nine minutes a day. Also apply Pointed Pressure Massage to the response areas for the sex glands and the stomach as shown in Chart 6 for nine minutes every three days. Put rubber bands on your first joint (nearest to the nail) of each finger as described under miscarriage.

NATURAL CHILD BIRTH

The idea that child birth has to be accompanied by the use of drugs, forceps, surgery, etc. is just not compatible with Nature's methods. If the mother has had proper nutrition and adequate pre-natal care, natural child birth may be had without drugs and their side effects. Complete books have been written on this subject, so we'll cover only the pertinent matters in the actual relief of pain and reduction of tension in the birth process.

There are several specific response areas for the reproductive organs. (See Charts 4, 5 and 6.) These should be massaged with pressure when the labor pains become severe. You should alternate putting rubber bands on first your fingers then your toes every half hour for nine minutes each.

In the moments just prior to birth, clasping the hands together and squeezing very hard will relax the entire body. While this doesn't relieve all the pain, it does keep it within a tolerable level and allows the mother to be conscious during the entire process. It also allows the baby to start life free from the effects of harmful drugs.

A CASE OF NATURAL CHILD BIRTH

Mrs. E. was advised by a mid-wife to clasp her hands tightly to relax her body and relieve the labor pains for her first child. She heeded the advice enroute to the hospital but was subsequently drugged, subjected to the surgeon's scalpel and the baby to forceps.

For her second child the use of natural methods afforded a completely natural birth. At the onset of labor she initiated the clasping of the hands for relaxation and relief of pain. As a result of this and natural living prior to delivery no drugs were needed.

With the resurgence of natural child birth today, the health of both mother and baby is improved in most cases.

NATURAL CHILD BIRTH

Mamie P. wanted to have her baby without drugs but was afraid the pain would be too much for her. Her cousin encouraged her to find a doctor who would help her achieve her goal of completely natural childbirth. Usually I try to start build-up exercises immediately following conception or, better yet, six months prior. Exercises designed to strengthen the muscles of the stomach and the pelvic region are very helpful in reducing the pain and trauma of birth.

TREATMENT:

Treatment during labor and birth is largely directed at sedation of the entire body so the natural processes can proceed without the tensions and forebodings which usually accompany the process. If this is done without drugs, everything proceeds more smoothly with less trauma and aftereffects.

For maximum benefits you should have two attendants helping apply pressure therapy plus the active participation of the mother-to-be during labor and birth. One attendant should be placing the rubber bands alternately on the first joint of the fingers and thumbs of both hands for nine minutes, then the feet for nine minutes. The other attendant should be applying pressure therapy with the thumb to the response areas for the uterus and ovaries as shown on Chart 6. The patient will be applying pressure to all zones by biting the tongue and clasping the hands together. Mamie cooperated fully and achieved her goal of completely natural childbirth with a minimum of pain and discomfort for her and all the advantages of a drugless birth for her baby.

chapter 13

Help For
The Asthmatic

The respiratory system is concerned with breathing, and consists of the nose and nasal cavities, the pharynx, and the larynx, the trachea and bronchi, and the lungs.

Air comes in through the nose and passes through the nasal cavities (passages) where it is warmed, moistened and filtered. Problems with the nose or nasal passages can be helped with pressure massage on the top of the foot just below the big toe as shown in Chart 6. Common problems that affect the nose or nasal passages include colds, hayfever, and nosebleeds. For colds, massage the response area for colds on the bottom of the feet just between the base of the big toe and the first toe as shown in Chart 2A and 2B. Hayfever is more associated with the endocrine glands so apply pressure massage to the response areas of the glands.

NOSEBLEEDS

A nose bleed can arise from a number of different causes but before your nose can bleed there must be a rupture of one or more of the many blood vessels that supply blood to the nose membranes. A lack of Vitamin C can cause unhealthy blood vessel walls and thus cause this to happen.

THE SINUSES

Associated with the nasal cavities are the paranasal sinuses, which are air-filled cavities in the bones of the head. All the sinuses open into the nasal cavities and consequently they frequently become infected with head colds. Many people suffer with sinus trouble and there is really no need for this. The sinuses can be cleared and kept clear with Pointed Pressure Massage and an addition of Vitamin C to your diet. Just apply pressure massage to the response area for the sinus just below the toes as shown in Chart 2A and 2B.

A CASE OF LONG-STANDING
SINUS TROUBLE CURED

Mr. D. suffered for years from a sinus condition which was extremely severe. He slept with a towel on his pillow to collect the yellow discharge every night. Believing there was nothing that could be done to stop this discharge and discomfort he continued to suffer not only with the annoying discharge but also from frequent colds and sore throats and had constant headaches.

After several years of this unnecessary discomfort Mr. D. came to my office in desperation. He felt that any relief

I could give him would be too good to be true. I began treating him with Pointed Pressure Massage on the response area for the sinuses all along the base of the toes on the bottom of the feet as shown in Chart 2A and 2B for immediate relief. In about nine minutes his headache was gone and he could feel his sinuses beginning to clear. I showed him the response areas for the sinuses on the foot (Charts 2A and 2B) and instructed him to massage the feet alternately for nine minutes each every third day until the tenderness was gone. I also explained the need for a saturated supplement of vitamin C. This is the addition of 1,000 to 2,000 mg of vitamin C a day. The amount should be spaced evenly over a 24 hour period, never taking more than 300 mg every four hours. Many people with sinus troubles need extra vitamin C and therefore this supplement must be added for the results of Pointed Pressure Massage to last.

Improvement began shortly and after six weeks of this self treatment the discharge was gone. Also the colds, sore throats and headaches were eliminated. By periodically continuing this pressure massage treatment and adding vitamin C to his diet he has been completely free from any sinus problems.

Most sinus sufferers are painfully aware that any relief at all is most welcome but few realize that this method can bring complete relief. Over a period of years, I have never seen a case of sinusitis that failed to disappear with this treatment. Whether it is acute or chronic, relief is only minutes away using pressure massage. Permanent relief has always necessitated an increase in vitamin C intake continuing indefinitely.

SORE THROATS

After the air has passed through the nasal passages it goes into the pharynx, a muscular membranous sac common to both food and air passages, then into the larynx at the upper end of the trachea. When breathing through the mouth, air also passes through the pharynx into the larynx. When a person has a sore throat the pharynx often becomes inflamed. Sore throats can be cleared up in nine minutes in many cases and even in the worst cases in 24 hours. When you have a sore throat apply pressure massage to the response areas for the throat on the hands and feet as shown in Charts 2A and 5. If the sore throat is more severe as in the case of strep throat, gargling with a vinegar solution of 60% water plus 40% vinegar every 15 minutes plus pressure massage on the response areas for nine minutes each will usually get rid of this in 24 hours.

THE LARYNX

As already stated the larynx is just below the pharynx. It is a cylindrical boxlike structure composed of nine cartilages. The most common of these cartilages are the epiglottis, the door-like entrance to the larynx which during swallowing acts as a lid to prevent food from going into the trachea or windpipe, and the thyroid cartilage which forms the prominence in the front of the neck and is commonly called the "Adam's Apple." The larynx is also called the voice box because it contains the vocal cords.

In swallowing, the entrance to the larynx, the glottis, is pulled up against the epiglottis so food cannot enter. However, if a foreign body does get in the larynx a coughing reflex is set off so as to expel it.

COUGHS

Persistent coughs such as with certain colds, hayfever, or whooping cough can be completely eliminated with pressure massage. There are several areas and ways to apply this pressure. First apply pressure on the tongue about 1/2 inch from the tip with your teeth. In other words bite down on it for nine minutes. Be sure and bite it for the full nine minutes but never longer than eleven minutes. Also apply pressure on the floor of the mouth beneath the tongue with a cotton tipped probe of some kind for seven to nine minutes daily. These two areas are the most common and will do the most good.

LARYNGITIS

Inflammation of the larynx is called laryngitis and results in a hoarseness or even a temporary loss of voice.

I recall the time when a young groom had laryngitis. He had been under the weather with the flu and developed laryngitis the day before his wedding. We were all at the wedding rehearsal and the minister was going over the ceremony and vows with the bride and groom asking them to repeat after him. It was then I learned he had laryngitis and could hardly talk. I advised him to stock up on vitamin C over the next 24 hours and to apply pressure massage on the area for the throat on the hands shown in Chart 5 continually for 30 minutes at a time several times during this 24 hour period. He started this and tried to get a good night's rest and sure enough the next evening at the wedding you could hear his vows loud and clear.

LUNGS

Extending from the larynx into the chest is the trachea or windpipe. It then divides into the right and left bronchi going into the corresponding lungs. The two lungs are not alike. The right lung has three lobes and the left has only two.

During breathing the size of the thoracic cavity is alternately increased and decreased. While inspiring the size of the chest cavity is increased. The ribs move up and out, increasing the front-to-back and the side-to-side diameters of the chest cavity. The diaphragm contracts increasing the head-to-foot diameter. The pressure inside the body is less than that outside the body or within the lungs. Consequently as the size of the chest cavity increases, air enters the lungs and expands them. Expiration is more passive. As the ribs lower and the diaphragm relaxes the air is forced out of the lungs. All the air in the lungs is not exchanged during respiration and there is always some residual air left in the lungs.

ASTHMA

Asthma is an ancient disease and is closely related to emotional states of the mind. It is an affection of the bronchial tubes characterized by difficulty in breathing, coughing and a feeling of constriction and suffocation. There is often violent gasping and wheezing in an asthmatic attack.

Causes of asthma include allergies to pets, pollen, some foods and dust. All of these while not critical in themselves may lead to asthma which can be very serious.

Have you ever seen a person struggling to get a little air into his lungs? The agony of the asthmatic's fight for air makes it one of man's most dreaded diseases. Many live in daily fear of suffocation and eventually die from its devastating effects. If you suffer from this dreaded disease then the story I am about to tell you may help you to help yourself with Pointed Pressure Massage.

A CASE OF ASTHMA DUE TO WHEAT DUST

Many cases of asthma develop from repeated bouts with colds, hayfever or prolonged exposure to some contaminating chemical or dust in the air. I knew a very young lad by the name of John who was spending his summers working in the wheat fields. Starting in Oklahoma where the first crops were ready for harvest he would follow the ripening crops north as far as the Canadian border. This exposed him to the dust of the wheat fields almost continually for 14 to 15 weeks.

The second summer he began to have a runny nose after about 6 weeks had passed. He thought he had a summer cold and failed to associate the problem with the dust. By the end of the summer he had begun having trouble breathing but his problem suddenly improved when he went back to school in the fall. The third summer he had his "summer cold" early and was having a mild asthma attack occasionally. By the end of the summer these attacks were becoming frequent and more severe. When he returned to school in the fall he continued to have attacks. He was subject to an attack any time and was becoming worried about permanent disability. Under thorough questioning and examination we determined that he had become allergic to dust particularly from the wheat field work in the summers.

A program of Pointed Pressure Massage twice weekly began to lessen the severity and frequency of the attacks. We found the response areas to the endocrine glands very tender at first and the response areas for the lungs and bronchial tubes shown in Chart 6 were very tender also. Within three months he was no longer having attacks and the wheezing during his breathing was gone. He decided to find summer employment away from the wheat fields the following summer and has had no return of his breathing difficulties. If you have similar problems in breathing you should immediately begin to massage the response areas for the lungs and bronchial tubes and those for the endocrine glands especially the pituitary, thyroid and adrenal glands. You should also try to eliminate any heavy exposure to an irritant such as dust or pollen.

As you can see with John's asthma, you must avoid all the things that you show an allergic reaction to and begin Pointed Pressure Massage to prevent asthmatic attacks. Since breathing is the key to life we must take every precaution to keep our respiratory system healthy.

ASTHMA

Larry D. began having problems breathing when he was a very young boy. By the time he was five, wheezing was his constant problem. A few times he was rushed to the hospital for oxygen. Allergy tests were not very helpful because he would react to almost anything.

TREATMENT:

Pressure therapy to the response area for the bronchial tubes and lungs as shown on Chart 6. Most asthmatics cannot tolerate the quantities of white sugar and white flour that the average person consumes. We began a program to restrict these items and formulate substitute items. For a child this is a problem.

LENGTH OF TREATMENT:

This usually requires many months of treatment so we instructed his parents in applying the pressure and gave him a check up every two months. After a year he was much improved. In two years his attacks were rare and very light. At this point they discontinued bringing him in for check-ups since the problem was gone as far as they were concerned. However they continued to watch the sugar and starch content in his diet.

chapter 14

Helping Restore Sight and Sound

The special sense organs are those concerned with the five senses. Those senses of taste, smell, sight, feeling and hearing.

As you know the tongue is an excellent indicator of the condition of health. Have you ever gone to a doctor who didn't ask you to let him look at your tongue? Many symptoms of disease clearly appear on the tongue. The normal tongue should be pink and clean. A discolored tongue, a coated tongue, or a dry, cracked tongue can mean a serious health problem.

Taste is perhaps one of the most important functions of the tongue. The organs of taste, located primarily on the tongue, are the taste buds. The four main tastes are sweet, sour, bitter and salty. Sweet and salty are tasted at the tip, sour is tasted along the sides and bitter is tasted at the base of the tongue.

Taste blindness, the inability to taste one or more of these tastes is common and hereditary. We all taste differently. The sense of taste is not just a luxury meant to give us pleasure when eating, but also it is a guide as to those foods that are nutritionally good for us.

A lot of taste blindness is due to a poor nerve supply. When this is the case, pressure massage on the response areas for the tongue as shown in Chart 5 will restore the proper nerve supply.

A TYPE OF TASTE BLINDNESS

Mrs. B. had been using too much salt on her food for over twenty-five years. She actually could taste very little except bitter and salty tastes. Unless everything was drowned in salt she thought it had no flavor. Her taste buds were dulled to the point of being able to detect only salt. She was having trouble with swollen ankles and pains in the chest and came with every other complaint possible in circulatory problems. Not once did she think her heavy salt intake was doing the damage in many ways. I found the response areas for the heart and circulation very tender. Of course I had to put her on a salt free diet for her other problems but I also knew it would allow me to restore her taste of food. We applied Pointed Pressure Massage to the response areas for her taste as well as her heart (Chart 5).

Improvement in the circulation was slow and by the time it was better so was the ability to enjoy the flavor of foods. Be sure you recognize this if you are a heavy salt eater. Begin at once to apply pressure massage to the response areas for the heart and the taste buds too. You can restore balance to your system and avoid serious consequences.

SMELL

The nerve cells for the sense of smell are found in, the upper part and back part of the nose. The lower part of the nose is used for breathing. Since smell is chemical in nature, anything that is smelled must be dissolved in the moist mucous membrane of the nose. The senses of smell and taste are closely related. If the nose is stopped up by a cold, sinus condition, or allergies, food does not taste as good. Smoking can also affect the sense of smell and taste. The loss of the sense of smell is often due to a poor nerve supply to the nerve cells for smell in the nose. This type of smell loss can be miraculously improved with pressure massage on the response areas for the nose. These are located all over the body. Chart 2A shows three of the most common areas.

TOUCH

The sense of feeling is felt all over the body. Located within the skin are specific receptors which are sensitive to the four basic sensations of pain, touch, temperature and pressure. Upon stimulation of a receptor, a nerve impulse is sent to the cerebral cortex of the brain where it is interpreted. Combinations of stimulations cause sensations such as burning, tickling, and itching. The brain must interpret the degree and combination of the stimulations for us to feel each sense properly. If the impulse that is sent to the brain is blocked in any way the sense of feeling can be lost or in many cases it will be jumbled because of the mixing of the impulses. This problem is found in a rare disease prevalent among Jewish children. When they get cut or scratched they cannot feel any sensation of pain. They do not go into shock as a normal child would. It can be very severe and seems to affect their speech as well.

THE EYE

The sense of sight is vital to all of us and we can not imagine its worth until we lose some of it. The organ of sight is the eye. It is a very complex little organ for its size. Since it is made of several important parts there are many problems which can affect the sense of sight if one part isn't functioning properly due to an injury, disease, etc.

The outer layer of the eye consists of a tough fibrous tissue forming the sclera which is the white of the eye, and the cornea, which is the transparent front part of the eye. The sclera is mostly protective in function but also serves as a place for the attachment of the muscles that move the eye. The cornea is a window for letting light rays into the eye and also the chief mechanism for converging the rays so they can be focused on the retina.

INFLAMMATION AND ULCERS

Problems with the sclera usually are in the form of an inflammation (scleritis). If the curvature of the cornea is not uniform, defective vision (astigmatism) results since all the light rays entering the eye are not brought to focus on the retina. Also scratches on the cornea may lead to ulcers and if neglected can produce blindness. Pressure massage on the response areas for the eyes as shown in Charts 3 and 5 will keep your sclera and cornea healthy and eliminate inflammation and ulcers. Exercising your eye muscles can many times help the problem of astigmatism also. An important exercise for the eyes will be explained a little later in the chapter under Cross-Eyes.

NIGHT BLINDNESS

The middle of the eye contains the blood vessels of the eyeball. The front part of the middle layer of the eye is the iris — a circular disc with a hole in the center of it called the pupil. This circular disc controls the size of the pupil according to the amount of light present. It protects the retina from being injured by too strong a light. Associated closely with the opening and closing of the pupil by the iris is the problem of night blindness. This is many times due to smoking but can be a nerve problem also. When this is the case, pressure massage on the response areas for the eye as shown in Charts 3 and 5 for nine minutes twice a week over a short period of time will do wonders.

BLOOD SHOT EYES

The story of blood shot eyes is another problem common in this area of the eye. It is usually due to too much alcohol or a vitamin deficiency. Addition of liver and other foods high in vitamin B as well as the vitamin itself along with pressure massage on the response areas for the eye will clear up those blood shot eyes and make them healthy again.

Immediately behind the iris and the pupil is the lens of the eye. It is a slightly yellow, transparent biconvex disc. There are ligaments on the sides to suspend it which are attached directly to the ciliary muscles of the eye. These muscles pull the lens so that it changes its shape for close and distant vision. Many people have to wear glasses at an early age to combat a weakness in the lens which prevents it from changing its shape correctly one way or the other. Often, these people might not have needed glasses really if they had applied Pointed Pressure Massage treatments to the eyes and exercised the eye muscles. The diet is also important in these cases. Carrots and sunflower seeds have been found to be fantastic medicine for the eyes.

CROSS-EYES

Cross-eyes are due to a weakness in the eye muscles. They can and should be corrected at an early age if possible.

First, by applying pressure massage to the response areas for the eyes on the hands and feet as shown in Charts 2A and 2B you can rejuvenate the whole eye area so that these muscles may begin to be strengthened. Then you must exercise your eyes daily by placing your index finger about one foot away from your face and moving it up and down and over and back as in a cross pattern as you follow its movement with your eyes without moving your head. Also follow the finger around in a circular motion. Do it with one eye then with the other; then with both eyes open and following it. This will strengthen the eye muscles and help to eliminate cross-eyes.

CATARACTS

In old age the lens tends to become opaque, a condition which can produce partial or complete blindness depending on the amount of light transmitted by the lens. This condition is called senile cataracts. Cataracts are also found in babies at birth (congenital cataracts) and at any age of a diabetic (diabetic cataracts). It is believed to accompany the degenerative changes in blood vessels that also occur in diabetics.

Cataracts need not be a serious problem. Many times they are due to vitamin deficiencies. By adding vitamins A, B, C, D and the trace minerals to your diet as well as applying Pointed Pressure Massage to the response areas for the eyes around the first joint of the index finger as shown in Chart 5 you can eliminate this potential threat of blindness completely.

CATARACTS ELIMINATED

Mrs. S. began having a slight blur in her vision and consulted me at the onset. When it was determined that cataracts were indeed being formed we began Pointed Pressure on the response areas for the eyes, Chart 5. With treatments twice weekly for six months we seemed to be losing the battle as the blur grew a little worse. Even though she was discouraged I insisted that we continue as I was sure we could eventually overcome the problem. Several weeks later the blur seemed to magically start to clear. We continued the pressure massage until all tenderness of the response area was gone. Her eyes are now normal and she doesn't require the thick glasses that surgery would have forced her to wear.

If you are afraid that cataracts may be developing, begin applying pressure massage to the tip of the second toe and continue to do this for nine minutes at least twice a week until all the tenderness is gone. You may very well save your most precious ability to see clearly without glasses.

The intermost layer of the eyeball is a nervous layer of tissue. It is called the retina and corresponds to the film of a camera. The retina contains the actual light-sensitive cells which are the rods and cones, as well as the outer nerve cells and a pigmented black layer. The pigmented layer absorbs light so that it will not be diffused and blur the image on the retina. The point where the optic nerve leaves the retina is called the blind spot because it is completely insensitive to light.

The eye then as well as the tongue is an important diagnostic organ. Through it the doctor can diagnose many diseases and common ailments. Some common problems that occur in the eye are: styes, weeping tear ducts, tired burning eyes and general eye troubles.

STYES

A stye is an inflammation of one or more of the sebaceous glands of the eyelid. It is usually caused by an irritation in the eyelid. They can be painful and should be done away with. Working the response areas for the eyes as shown in Chart 5 and bathing the eyes in hot moist tea leaves will clear them up in no time.

WEEPING TEAR DUCTS

Weeping tear ducts which cause the eyes to water all the time are usually due to irritants in the air. If this is a problem with your eyes, apply pressure massage to the response areas on the lower knuckle joint of the index finger for the eye as shown in Chart 2A.

TIRED, BURNING EYES

There are many things that can tire and cause burning in the eyes. Too much reading, close focusing, driving, etc. will tire the eyes and the best treatment for this is to rest those eyes. If you have a lot of reading, take short breaks where you can refocus your eyes. Smog, smoke, dust and dirt can cause burning in the eyes. We must protect our eyes from these pollutants. When these things cause problems you should wash your eyes with clear warm water and then apply pressure massage to the response areas on the index fingers as shown also in Chart 5 for nine minutes. This will relax the eyes.

GENERAL

Any general problems with the eyes can be relieved with Pointed Pressure Massage applied to the response areas to the eyes (Chart 5) and to the kidneys as shown in Chart 2B. If your kidneys are not working properly this can often affect your eyes so working their response areas will help both the kidneys as well as the eyes.

THE EAR

The sense of hearing is a very vital and necessary sense. The organ of hearing and balance is the ear. It consists of the outer ear, middle ear, and inner ear. The tympanic membrane, or ear drum as it is commonly called, separates the outer ear from the middle. Within the middle ear is a tube that communicates with the nasal cavity and nose which is called the eustachian tube. The function of the eustachian tube is to equalize the air pressure on each side of the ear drum. That is to equalize the pressure in the middle ear with that of the external atmosphere in the outer ear. This tube also serves as a route for the spread of infection from the nose, for example a bad head cold, to the middle ear.

The inner ear is where the true organs of hearing and balance are. The organs of corti within the cochlea of the inner ear have hair cells which when stimulated create nerve impulses which are carried to the brain, where they are recognized as sounds. The semicircular canals also in the inner ear are the organs of balance. Here also hair cells are stimulated which set up nerve impulses important in maintaining the dynamic equilibrium of the body.

DEAFNESS

I guess the worst problem that occurs in the ears is deafness. Usually if you are going deaf it continues to get worse and does not go away as an earache would. Deafness can be caused by an impacted wisdom tooth, catarrh, thickening of the membranes of the inner ear (otosclerosis) and hardened ear wax. If the problem is hardened ear wax, ear drops can be used to remove the wax and probably will need to be used again as the wax developes and hardens again. Also, if the problem is an impacted wisdom tooth, then the tooth should be extracted immediately before it causes more damage.

Pressure massage can be used very effectively with many cases of deafness. There are several places and methods to apply the pressure massage needed. First I would recommend thoroughly massaging the response areas for the ears on the feet as shown in Charts 2A and 2B. Then massage the response areas for the ears on the joints of the 3rd, 4th and 5th fingers of the hands. These are probably the easiest areas to work on but there are other ones that do as much or more good. The first one is the gum area in back of the wisdom teeth. It is harder to apply pressure here in the normal manner so we suggest getting a rubber eraser that will fit into the area and biting down on it with the gums for nine minutes every third day. Secondly the tongue has response areas for many organs and their problems. By applying pressure massage on it you can clear up many acute as well as chronic problems. Here is how it is done. First stick out your tongue about 1/2 inch. Then bite down on it very firmly with your teeth for nine minutes. Be careful not to bit down too hard and continue the bite for the full nine minutes for the best results. NEVER go longer than 11 minutes at one time. Generally this method should be done once every three days but can be done up to three times a day in acute cases.

EAR WAX CAN CAUSE DEAFNESS

Mr. P.'s hearing was gradually deteriorating even though he had made repeated attempts to find professional help for the problem. Every one gave him the same answer "There is nothing we can do for you because we can't find a reason for the loss of hearing." Every part of the ear seemed to be normal but nonetheless he was loosing his hearing.

In locating the cause we found there was a very small but perceptible improvement each time a different specialist had examined him. This improvement was subsequently lost within a few days following each visit. He remembered that they washed out his ears at each visit but attached no significance to this. He always seemed to have a lot of wax in his ears but not enough to block the passages. There was however, enough wax ever present to cause pressure on the lining of the ear. This was just enough to block some nerve supply to the brain centers.

We found the response areas to the ears very tender and began applying pressure massage to these areas immediately. In a few weeks the overproduction of wax in the ear was curtailed and the hearing response began to return. His hearing is now normal and will remain so because the cause of the problem has been removed.

EARACHES

Earaches are common problems today, not only with children but also with many adults. They need not be a problem with pressure massage. Just apply pressure massage to the response areas for the ears for nine minutes at a time. Sometimes it is helpful to apply pressure massage with a wooden clothes pin on the tip of the ring finger for nine minutes. Also pulling down and forward on the lobe of the ear for nine minutes will relieve the pain of an earache many times.

RINGING EARS

Tinnitus, ringing in the ears, can be caused by a wax build-up in the ear, perforations of the tympanic membrane, fluid in the middle ear or an impacted wisdom tooth. Anything that causes a nerve blocking can cause ringing ears. The treatment is very similar to that for deafness.

RINGING EARS DUE TO
AN IMPACTED WISDOM TOOTH

Mrs. J. was about to resign her position as the head of the language department in her school because of a hearing problem which was beginning to affect her concentration.

She was afraid it would progressively get worse and drive her out of her mind.

An examination revealed an extreme tenderness in the response areas for the ear shown in Chart 2A and 2B. If you will study these Charts carefully you will find that the teeth response areas are in the same zone as the ear. You will notice that the response area for the wisdom tooth falls in the zone with the ring finger on Chart 2.

Many hearing problems are a result of a nerve blocking due to tooth impaction or crowded teeth. In this case the response areas for the wisdom tooth were also extremely tender indicating that there was an underlying tooth condition which was involved in the hearing problem.

I advised her to see her dentist for the removal of the wisdom tooth before we attempted to restore the nerve supply to the ear. She didn't like the idea of having the tooth removed so we tried to restore the nerve supply with Pointed Pressure Massage. After three weeks of treatment with only a slight improvement she agreed to see her dentist. The tooth was definitely impacted and needed to be removed, however, the dentist could not agree that this was connected to the hearing problem.

Several weeks after the tooth had been removed she returned to my office. The ringing in her ears was only slightly improved by the removal of the tooth.

We began to apply Pointed Pressure Massage to the response areas for the ear and for the teeth as well. In the third week of treatment she began to notice the improvement she had been hoping for. At the end of the eighth week all ringing had ceased and she was able to resume her normal teaching routine.

TINNITIS

Ms. S. began having a ringing noise in her ear during her second year of teaching. By the end of the year it was so annoying she was ready to quit teaching, having been unable to find any medical answer to her problem. When she became afraid it was altering her mental outlook she was ready to try anything.

TREATMENT:

Pointed Pressure Therapy on the four zones as shown on Charts 1, 2A and 2B, and 3.

LENGTH OF TREATMENT:

Four weeks of formal treatments during which time I applied pointed pressure to the response area on the back as shown on Chart 5 for nine minutes twice weekly. I instructed her to wrap a rubber band on the first joint of the fourth toe of each foot, three times weekly for nine minutes and on alternate days the same thing on the fourth finger. She continued the rubber band therapy for another four weeks until all ringing stopped. She has regained her good mental outlook and has experienced no return of the ringing after many years.

chapter 15

Quick Relief
For Minor Ailments

Little Johnny knew instinctively how to obtain immediate relief from teething pain or just plain anxiety. Since early childhood he sucked his thumb regularly. This caused his upper teeth to protrude so far that his appearance was causing the other kids to ridicule him. He was a nervous type of child anyway and was becoming more emotionally upset every day. All attempts to find the cause or a way to correct the problem had failed.

When his parents brought him to my office for an examination he was certainly a pathetic young lad. I had difficulty in calming him enough to make a complete evaluation of his trouble. I did finally discover a severe subluxation of the 3rd cervical vertebrae. Further interrogation revealed he had fallen on his head and shoulder when he was about a year old. He was treated for a cut on the head at that time but no X-rays were taken. No subsequent examination had revealed this spinal problem.

I always check for cervical misalignment in any nervous condition because this is the problem in many cases. Thumb-sucking is generally present in the young when there is any feeling of uneasiness or pain. It is one of the most misunderstood activities in children. This sucking instinct offers to the child a means of applying Pointed Pressure Massage for his anxiety and or pain as the case may be. Without knowing what he is doing he is obtaining the only relief available. Sucking the thumb when observed very closely is actually applying pressure to the lower lip and to the roof of the mouth. While this pressure is not great enough to effect a cure for a specific problem such as a subluxated vertebrae, it does give a general relaxation and relief of pain.

By applying Pointed Pressure Massage to the response area for the cervical section of the spine as shown in Chart 2A we were able to correct the subluxation in about four weeks. The change in the lad's personality was noticeable immediately when he stopped sucking his thumb. I suggested a visit to the dentist for corrective braces now that he had stopped the thumbsucking. In a year the braces had corrected most of the malformation of the teeth and he was a happy, well-adjusted lad.

TWITCH ON LIP

Evidence of this tranquilizing effect of pressure massage can be seen in the animal world. Everyone has seen the mother cat pick her young up by the nape of the neck and carry them about. The kitten is rendered immobile and free of pain in this specialized case of Pointed Pressure Massage. Similarly those familiar with the raising of horses will recognize the specialized application of Pointed Pressure Massage by placing a twitch on the upper lip of a horse. When treating an injured horse all pain can be removed by placing a twitch on the upper lip of the horse and tightening it while treating the injury.

This type of immediate relief can be had in many common problems such as those that occur in the following examples.

HEADACHES

You may relieve that sudden headache by pressing on your forehead about one half inch above the bridge of the nose for nine minutes. Keep a rolling type of heavy pressure massage on this area and you will be able to relieve most headaches, in a natural way without damaging your health with drugs. Another quick way to relieve a headache is to bite your tongue. You do this by sticking your tongue out about a half inch and biting down on it gently but firmly for nine minutes. Be sure to keep constant pressure on the tongue through the nine minutes. Never go longer than eleven minutes.

A third way to relieve a headache in about nine minutes is to put rubber bands on your fingers at the first joint (one nearest the nail). Be sure they are on tight and leave them on for nine minutes. It should hurt a little and the ends of the fingers should turn red then purplish.

TEMPORARY CONSTIPATION

If you have only an occasional bout with constipation you may get immediate relief without a laxative. By applying Pointed Pressure Massage to the center of your chin just above the jaw bone and below the lower lip in the little groove, you will have a completely normal evacuation of tne bowels in less than fifteen minutes. For chronic constipation you will need to correct your living habits as described in the chapter on digestion.

STIFF NECK

If you occasionally are bothered by a stiff neck, you can have relief in minutes by pressure massage on the bottom of your foot just below the base of the little toe. This usually needs to be repeated approximately three times a day for complete relief but will give you immediate relief in a few minutes.

SORE THROAT

Suffering with a sore throat for three or four days is a very miserable period of time. In a few minutes you can relieve the rawness by gargling with a solution of weak vinegar — usually a 50/50 mixture. After the initial gargling, pressure massage between the thumb and the first finger at the base of the thumb will keep the soreness at a tolerable level. In most cases complete relief is available in 24 hours.

GAS

When there is no anti-acid available you may want to get immediate relief by massaging the center of the bottom of the foot for nine minutes. This will usually free trapped gas so it can be expelled. This is one way to prevent problems with the appendix. It is very unwise to keep trapped gas in the system since this can cause the appendix to rupture.

HICCOUGHS

Whether your hiccough problem is occasional or chronic you may end the problem by applying Pointed Pressure Massage to the center of the bottom of the foot. Many people have obtained relief when all other attempts have failed including surgery. It will usually take nine minutes of very vigorous massage to get results. If you don't get results it is because you haven't been vigorous enough or applied pressure long enough.

EARACHE

Don't take the chance of inserting anything smaller than your elbow in your ear. An earache may be caused by several different things. If there is something in the ear you should consult your physician immediately but if it is a periodic complaint associated with wind or cold you should be able to get immediate relief by massaging the tip of the toe next to your little toe. Should the pain continue expert assistance should be obtained immediately.

SINUS

For that change of weather or altitude type of sinus pressure which is so unbearable you can get quick relief by applying pressure massage to the area at the base of the three smaller toes on each foot. This will open the sinus passages up so the pressure can be equalized and thus give you quick relief.

MIGRAINE HEADACHE

Ms. K. lived in fear of the sure return of her unwanted headache that put her in bed for two to three days.

Migraine headache is sometimes attributed to a nervous problem which occurs periodically. There is some evidence of a genetic trait but no proof.

The word migraine comes from a French word meaning "one side of the head" but this does not mean the headache is always on one side or the other for it often occurs over the entire head. Sometimes it lasts for days. The torture of these headaches is unbelievable for someone who has not experi-

enced them. Anyone should seek professional help if troubled
with migraine headaches because they can be a symptom of a
more serious disorder such as a tumor on the brain. In this case
we did a complete "work up" before concluding that there was
no pathological condition causing them, other than the weakened condition of the pancreas. Curtailing sweets, chocolate
and white flour products always helps when there is a sugar imbalance. I have seen cases where white sugar was the lone problem in the case of migraine.

If little Jr. or Susie throw many tantrums, watch the white
sugar intake — children have headaches and emotional problems from this. If the pancreas is already weakened they may
require pressure therapy to correct the problem.

TREATMENT FOR MS. K:

Pointed Pressure Therapy applied to the forehead as
shown on Chart 4. Since many who suffer from migraine
headaches, suffer from poor sugar balance caused by problems with the Islets of Langerhans, we usually find the response area on Chart 2B for the pancreas very sore — such
was the case here.

LENGTH OF TREATMENT:

Nine minutes pressure on each of these points twice weekly for three months.

Recovery came slowly — from weekly headaches to none
at the end of three months.

After five years, no reoccurrence and no fear of the ter-
rible pain which aspirin or other headache remedies could help.

HICCOUGHS

Several years ago I picked up the newspaper and read a
story with the following title "Marine Stops Hiccoughs for
Hospitalized Man." A man had been exhausted by a seige of
hiccoughs that had plagued him night and day for several days.

The doctor had tried everything without success and was considering an operation in an attempt to stop the seige before it killed him.

When the marine heard of the poor fellow's problem, he volunteered to come to the hospital and try to help him by rubbing the bottom of his foot.

TREATMENT:

Even though the doctors were skeptical and brushed the thought aside as ridiculous, the man's family were not so sure that this shouldn't be tried — in fact they insisted the marine come to the hospital and try in spite of the skeptics. The marine came to the man's bedside and began pressure therapy on the bottom of the foot.

LENGTH OF TREATMENT:

Within ten minutes the spasms were gone and the man was resting. He continued applying the pressure for nearly half an hour and then told the family and doctors to do some more if the problem returned. It did not return so the patient was released the next day after having had a good night's sleep.

STIFF NECK

Mrs. C. had been unable to turn her head to the right for several years following a severe bump on the head. She had bent over to move a calf in the barn and raised up — forgetting there was a beam above her. The blow nearly made her unconscious but she quickly revived and except for the bump on the head she forgot it. The next day she realized she couldn't turn her head to the right. She refused to see a chiropractor because she was afraid he would "break her neck." The discomfort grew gradually worse as the years went by and finally she heard of a new doctor in town that pinched the bottom of the foot for back trouble. She came to me and I told her I believed I could help her.

TREATMENT:

Pointed Pressure Therapy for the response areas on the bottom of the foot as shown on Charts 2A and 2B for nine minutes continuing for three weeks. At the end of three weeks the movement was nearly back to normal so we discontinued the formal treatments. I asked her to continue the massage for herself for another month, which she did. Her return check-up revealed no problem in the neck area.

Many people have problems in the neck area that they do not recognize because they are only slightly uncomfortable. What they do not realize is that some function of the body is being hampered because of a pinched nerve or suluxated vertebrae. Numerous school children receive bumps on the head which are the beginnings of health problems. Don't assume that the neighbor boy hitting your boy on the head with a school-book is just going to give him a temporary headache. It might injure him very badly. Insist on an examination any time the bump is on the head.

INDEX